first place
4health
Bible Study Series

walking in
grace

Published by Gospel Light
Ventura, California, U.S.A.
www.gospellight.com
Printed in the U.S.A.

Library of Congress Cataloging-in-Publication Data
First Place 4 Health Bible study series : walking in grace.
p. cm.
ISBN 978-0-8307-5490-8 (trade paper)
1. Grace (Theology)—Biblical teaching—Textbooks. 2. Christian life—Biblical
teaching—Textbooks. I. First Place 4 Health (Organization) II. Title: Walking
in grace.
BS680.G7F57 2010
234.07—dc22
2010013198

Rights for publishing this book outside the U.S.A. or in non-English
languages are administered by Gospel Light Worldwide, an international
not-for-profit ministry. For additional information, please visit
www.glww.org, email info@glww.org, or write to Gospel Light Worldwide,
1957 Eastman Avenue, Ventura, CA 93003, U.S.A.

To order copies of this book and other Gospel Light products in bulk
quantities, please contact us at 1-800-446-7735.

contents

BIBLE STUDIES

ADDITIONAL MATERIALS

foreword

My introduction to Bible study came when I joined First Place in March 1981. I had been attending church since I was a small child, but the extent of my study of the Bible had been reading my Sunday School quarterly on Saturday night. On Sunday morning, I would listen to my Sunday School teacher as she taught God's Word to me. During the worship service, I would listen to our pastor as he taught God's Word to me. Frankly, the idea of digging out the truths of the Bible for myself had never entered my mind.

Perhaps you are right where I was back in 1981. If so, you are in for a blessing you never dreamed possible. As you start studying the truths of the Bible for yourself through the First Place 4 Health Bible studies, you will see God begin to open your understanding of His Word.

Almost every First Place 4 Health member I have talked with about the program says, "The weight loss is wonderful, but the most important thing I have received from my association with First Place 4 Health is learning to study God's Word." The First Place 4 Health Bible studies are designed to be done on a daily basis. As you work through each day's study (which will take 15 to 20 minutes to complete), you will be discovering the deep truths of God's Word. A part of each week's study will also include a Bible memory verse for the week.

There are many in-depth Bible studies on the market. The First Place 4 Health Bible studies are not designed for the purpose of in-depth study, but are designed to be used in conjunction with the rest of the program to bring balance into your life. Our desire is for each member to begin having a personal quiet time with God each day. This time alone with God should include a time of prayer, Bible reading and Bible study. Having a quiet time is a daily discipline that will bring the rich rewards of balance, which is something we all need.

God bless you as you begin this exciting journey toward a balanced life. God will richly bless your efforts to give Him first place in your life. Remember Matthew 6:33: "But seek first his kingdom and his righteousness, and all these things will be given to you as well."

Carole Lewis, First Place 4 Health National Director

introduction

First Place 4 Health is a Christ-centered health program that emphasizes balance in the physical, mental, emotional and spiritual areas of life. The First Place 4 Health program is meant to be a daily process. As we learn to keep Christ first in our lives, we will find that He is the One who satisfies our hunger and our every need.

This Bible study is designed to be used in conjunction with the First Place 4 Health program but can be beneficial for anyone interested in obtaining a balanced lifestyle. The Bible study has been created in a five-day format, with the last two days reserved for reflection on the material studied. Keep in mind that the ultimate goal of studying the Bible is not only for knowledge but also for application and a changed life. Don't feel anxious if you can't seem to find the *correct* answer. Many times, the Word will speak differently to different people, depending on where they are in their walk with God and the season of life they are experiencing. Be prepared to discuss with your fellow First Place 4 Health members what you learned that week through your study.

There are some additional components included with this study that will be helpful as you pursue the goal of giving Christ first place in every area of your life:

- **Group Prayer Request Form:** This form is at the end of each week's study. You can use this to record any special requests that might be given in class.

- **Leader Discussion Guide:** This discussion guide is provided to help the First Place 4 Health leader guide a group through this Bible study. It includes ideas for facilitating a First Place 4 Health class discussion for each week of the Bible study.

- **Two Weeks of Menu Plans with Recipes:** There are 14 days of meals, and all are interchangeable. Each day totals 1,400 to 1,500 calories and includes snacks. Instructions are given for those who need more calories. An accompanying grocery list includes items needed for each week of meals.

- **First Place 4 Health Member Survey:** Fill this out and bring it to your first meeting. This information will help your leader know your interests and talents.

- **Personal Weight and Measurement Record:** Use this form to keep a record of your weight loss. Record any loss or gain on the chart after the weigh-in at each week's meeting.

- **Weekly Prayer Partner Forms:** Fill out this form before class and place it into a basket during the class meeting. After class, you will draw out a prayer request form, and this will be your prayer partner for the week. Try to call or email the person sometime before the next class meeting to encourage that person.

- **Live It Trackers:** Your Live It Tracker is to be completed at home and turned in to your leader at your weekly First Place 4 Health meeting. The Tracker is designed to help you practice mindfulness and stay accountable with regard to your eating and exercise habits. Step-by-step instructions for how to use the Live It Tracker are provided in the *Member's Guide*.

- **Let's Count Our Miles!** A worthy goal we encourage is for you to complete 100 miles of exercise during your 12 weeks in First Place 4 Health. There are many activities listed on pages 255-256 that count toward your goal of 100 miles. When you complete a mile of activity, mark off the box listed on the Hundred Mile Club chart located on the inside of the back cover.

- **Scripture Memory Cards:** These cards have been designed so you can use them while exercising. It is suggested that you punch a hole in the upper left corner and place the cards on a ring. You may want to take the cards in the car or to work so you can practice each week's Scripture memory verse throughout the day.

- **Scripture Memory CD:** All 10 Scripture memory verses have been put to music at an exercise tempo in the CD at the back of this study. Use this CD when exercising or even when you are just driving in your car. The words of Scripture are often easier to memorize when accompanied by music.

welcome to
walking in grace

At your first group meeting for this session of First Place 4 Health, you will meet your fellow members, get an overview of your materials and find out what you can expect at weekly meetings. The majority of your class time will be spent learning about the four-sided person concept, the Live It Food Plan, and how change begins from the inside out. You will also have a chance to ask any questions about how to get the most out of First Place 4 Health. If possible, complete the Member Survey on page 205 before your first group meeting. The information that you give will help your leader tailor the next 12 weeks to the needs of the whole group.

Each weekly meeting begins with a weigh-in for members. This will allow you to track your progress over the 12-week session. Your Week One weigh-in/measurement will establish a baseline of comparison so that you can set healthy goals for this session. If you are apprehensive about weighing in every week, talk with your group leader about your concerns. He or she will have some options for you to consider that will make the weigh-in activity encouraging rather than stressful.

The day after your first meeting, begin Week Two of this Bible study. This session, you and your group will examine God's grace, given to help you live life to the fullest every day. As you open yourself to the truth of Scripture and share your hopes and struggles with the members of your group during the next 12 weeks, you'll find yourself becoming the healthy child of God you are designed to be!

3.2-17

Week Two

gift of grace

SCRIPTURE MEMORY VERSE
Now the Lord is the Spirit, and where the Spirit of the Lord is there is freedom.
2 CORINTHIANS 3:17

Imagine receiving a beautiful gift tied with a golden bow—and it's not even your birthday or Christmas! Someone who loves you has chosen to give you a special gift. This gift is better than new clothes that will eventually wear out, better than items that rust or get used up. More than a dazzling piece of jewelry that is worn only on the outside, this gift brings a sparkle within your heart that radiates outward to everyone around you.

The gift is God's grace, and He gives it generously. Grace frees us from the struggle of doing everything on our own. Willpower is difficult in a world of temptation—a world filled with sweets and savory foods. God knows our need for something more than our own power and offers His grace to overcome challenges and free us to live a healthy, balanced life. This week, we will look at God's wonderful gift of grace and at how it frees us to change.

Day 1 ENOUGH GRACE

Gracious God, You want to free me from worry and temptation.
I want Your grace, the help I don't deserve, to be with me today. Amen.

In the opening greeting of his second letter to the Corinthians, the apostle Paul used the phrase "grace and peace to you from God our Father and the Lord Jesus Christ" (2 Corinthians 1:2). In fact, Paul opened and closed almost every letter he wrote with the blessing "grace to you." It seems clear that Paul had discovered the secret to beginning and ending his thoughts and days centered on receiving God's grace.

Yet, Paul also struggled with something he called a "thorn in the flesh." (We don't know if his problem was physical, mental, spiritual or emotional; Paul did not give us the details.) He pleaded with God three times to take away his problem, but God did not take it away. Instead, He spoke wise words about how His grace would give Paul the strength he needed for enduring the struggle.

Today we will look at how God's grace gives people strength and undeserved help when they face difficult circumstances.

Turn in your Bible to 2 Corinthians 12:7-10. What reason did Paul give for God giving him a thorn in the flesh?

To keep me from conceited

What did Paul ask God to do about the problem? How hard and often did he ask for help?

3 times take away this problems

How did God answer Paul? How does His answer apply to you?

God's grace is sufficient

3-9-17

Notice that God did not take away the problem even when Paul pleaded repeatedly. At the end of verse 9, Paul "boasts" (or "glories" in some translations) in his weakness. What is the reason?

so that Christs power may rest on me

The word "grace" in the New Testament is the Greek word *charis*. It is used to refer to the undeserved kindness of God or a gift from God, and throughout the New Testament it denotes God's own empowering, enabling presence with us through the Holy Spirit (see Acts 4:33; Romans 12:6; 1 Corinthians 15:10; Hebrews 10:29). The Greek word in 2 Corinthians 12:9 for "rest upon me" in the verse means to cover, as a tabernacle or tent. Like Paul's thorn in the flesh, God covers our weaknesses with the power of His grace. How did Paul feel about his problem after God answered him (see verse 10)?

That is why for Christ sake, I delight in weaknesses, in insults, in hardship, in persecutions, in difficulties. For when I am weak then I am strong

God didn't take away Paul's thorn in the flesh, but His grace gave him strength to continue. In the First Place 4 Health journey, many of us struggle to achieve and maintain healthy weight and a strong, fit body . . . a thorny problem, indeed! Yet the program speaks of progress, not perfection. That means learning to forgive yourself for weakness or failure instead of letting guilt consume you and giving up. Do you need to let go of any guilt now, accepting God's grace as a cover for your weaknesses?

Once we have accepted God's grace and forgiveness for our shortcomings, He offers His help and strength for our continuing growth. Reflect on the memory verse and the idea of freedom from struggles. Do you need freedom from worry, temptations, or guilt through God's helping grace?

_____

_____

_____

_____

Gracious Father, may Your grace be with me today. Guide me in my choices. May Your grace free me from temptations that cause me to stumble. Amen.

3-15-17

FREEDOM OF GRACE

Day 2

Gracious Father, help me learn to rely on Your grace daily and to lean on the group of friends in First Place 4 Health who are walking with me. Amen.

Paul spent time in jail, where he received beatings and other harsh treatment for his faith. But he never gave up or let the chains imprison his spirit. He prayed with joy because his friends remained in his heart and shared in God's grace with him. God's grace sustained him and helped him focus not on his problems, but on his connection to other Christians. God's grace, enough for you each day, can also bring you closer with other Christians and help you experience real freedom.

Today we will study how God's grace helps us fellowship with other Christians despite our circumstances and changes our focus from self to unity with others in Christ.

Read Philippians 1:1-7. What is the source of grace and peace?

from God our Father and the Lord Jesus Christ

How did praying for and partnering with others make Paul feel?

joyful & confident

What will happen to the good work God has begun in you? How can other believers be a part of it?

that we might carry it on to completion we can share in God's grace

Whether Paul was in chains or not, he was free within his heart. How is this an example of freedom in grace? What do you and other believers share with Paul?

God's grace

Read Philippians 4:23. Where does it say the grace of peace should be? What would this look like in your life?

be with your spirit

In Philippians 1:2, Paul greeted people with the desire for them to receive God's grace. How might you express a desire for others to have God's grace without sounding preachy? How can others challenge you to receive more of God's grace?

we need to be open to others comment as we learn more from each other and at bible study

We sometimes call praying before meals "saying grace." Each time before you eat this week, stop to ask for God's grace to help you make good nutritious choices. In our study today we noted that Paul expressed confidence that God who began a good work in you will carry it to completion. How does this help you know that God will help you complete the work you have begun with First Place 4 Health?

God is alway there for us if we only ask.

Thank You, gracious Lord, for giving me grace and friends to help me daily make better choices. Amen.

3-30.17

PAUL, CHANGED BY GRACE

Day 3

Gracious Father, thank You for Your grace that is enough for today. I trust that You will help me live with better choices for a healthy lifestyle. Amen.

Paul attributed many changes in his life to God's grace. He changed from persecuting Christians to following Jesus and being willing to suffer persecution. Today we'll look at Paul's testimony of how grace worked in his life. His powerful witness helps us know that grace is real and can make a difference in our lives.

A personal endorsement and testimony are powerful and make us see possibilities for our own lives. Many people come to First Place 4 Health because of the testimony of a friend. Have you met people changed by the program? Seeing evidence in someone's life helps us trust that the program will work.

Beyond outward appearance and better health, many people in First Place 4 Health are changed within and have more joy in life. This comes from God's grace at work in them. Reflect on how you and others in your First Place 4 Health group are changing for the better through God's grace.

Read 1 Timothy 1:12-16. What were Paul's past faults (see verse 13)?

a liar, persecuted - violent man

According to verse 12, how did Jesus view Paul?

gave him strength and appointed him to Jesus service

The key to all the change in Paul's life is noted in verse 14. What happened to Paul to change him so dramatically?

The grace of God was poured out on him

4-6-17

Paul called himself "the worst of sinners." He persecuted the early Christians and even oversaw the execution of one named Stephen (see Acts 7:55–8:1). Yet God reached out and changed Paul (see Acts 9:1-19). He turned from hating Christians to being a believer, from persecuting to being persecuted. Even more, Paul changed inside to become a man contented in all circumstances. Read Philippians 4:11-13. What did Paul learn that helped him to be content?

he could do everything through our God who gave him strength

Read Philippians 4:4-8. List the practical tips Paul gave for focusing our minds on positive thoughts and giving worries to God.

whatever is true, noble, right, pure, lovely admirable, excellent praise worthy

We can choose to rejoice in God and give Him our worries in prayer, rather than dwelling on our difficult circumstances. Make a list of some positive thoughts to dwell on this week. Carry the list with you and pull it out when you are feeling overwhelmed by your difficulties.

The weather is getting nicer
Easter Sunday   Aarons birthday
our trip to Co.
Ellie & kids coming up.

In Philippians, Paul 4:6 urges us to take our anxieties and give them to God in prayer with thanksgiving. Write a prayer about your worries and then offer them to God, thanking Him that His grace is sufficient for you.

Lord, what is upmost in our minds
is our country. Please help us get turned
around in our thinking. Please keep
us all safe. Thank You.   Amen

Ask God to help you let go of the past. You are under His grace now, not under the past. You are free to make new choices, to serve God and to learn to be content. Combining prayer with thanksgiving helps us to trust God for the answers. With thanks, we remember that God listens to and walks with us, offering us abundant grace to face whatever lies ahead.

> *Father, pour out Your grace on me abundantly. Help me to be content on the inside and instruct me in the knowledge I need for living a godly life. Amen.*

4-27-17

A LIFE OF GRACE

Day 4

> *God, You created me and love me. You have been gracious to pour out Your grace on me. Give me the power of Your grace to continue changing. Amen.*

Paul understood the power of God's grace to help us live godly lives, and he shared about this in a letter to his friend Titus. God wants you to understand the amazing power of His grace. It will help you change and turn away from worldly desires. Today we will look at how grace can impact our choices to enable us to change and live more godly lives.

Read Titus 2:11-15. Who can receive God's grace (see verse 11) and what can it help us do (see verse 12)?

all men (everyone)

a teaches us to say no to ungodliness
& worldly passion - to live self controlled
upright & godly lives

God's grace guides us to turn from worldly desires. As we receive grace, we can make better choices. We can say no to worldly desire for sweets, fatty foods or other temptations. It gives us self-control to resist cravings. And self-control helps us say yes to godly choices of exercise, healthy foods and prayer. It may seem hard to just say no. That's because we often dwell on the negative and our desire for it. Yet God offers us new thoughts to help us turn our mind from the worldly desires.

"Upright life" could also be translated "sensible life," a life lived righteously and with wisdom. Thus, living with grace trains us to live wisely and virtuously in a way that honors God. It's living in the presence of God and making choices that He would approve. Verses 13-15 tell us more about the upright way of life. What do we wait for?

the blessed hope the glorious appearing
of our great God & Savior Jesus Christ

Our hope is something positive to hold on to as we resolve not to continue in unhealthy choices. We have the hope of the coming of Jesus. So, don't just say "No." Say "No thanks, I have something better to do with my time. I can look toward Jesus for my happiness and satisfaction. I don't need momentary pleasures." What does God purify us for, and how does it change us (see verse 14)?

to redeem us from all wickedness & to purify us His very own people

Read Titus 3:1-2. What are some ways to do what is good?

to slander no one - to be peaceable & considerate and to show true humility toward all men

God's grace changes us on the inside. Part of that change causes us to be zealous, eager to show God our love in how we treat other people. What are some ways you can show your love for God in how you treat the members of your First Place 4 Health group?

always listen to their concerns, be willing to help any way I can. encourage them.

How does First Place 4 Health help you live in a way that pleases God?

God has lead me to people that I can talk to and ask question and I can share in their lives as well as they can share in mine

Gracious Father, make me eager to please You. Thank You for Your abundant grace in my life that has freed me to make better choices and lead a more balanced life. Amen.

Day
5

GRACE AND COMPASSION

Dear Lord, it's amazing to know that You pour out grace every day. Help me to understand the depth of Your grace. Amen.

God's grace helped Paul live a more godly life and taught him to treat other people with compassion. Having compassion means to have passion with or to suffer with someone. Today we will look at passages in Psalms about the graciousness and compassion of God, who teaches us how to be compassionate toward others.

Read Psalm 84:11. What does God give? What does He not withhold from those who walk uprightly with Him?

he bestows favor & honor
no good thing does He withhold

Now turn to Psalm 111:4-10. How does verse 4 describe God?

gracious - Loving
compassionate

6, 7-6
29 What are specific works mentioned in Psalm 111 that God has done to show His grace and compassion?

giving them land
the works of His hand are faithful & Just
they are steadfast forever

What promises do you find in the psalm?

His promises are steadfast

The psalm starts with praising God's simple act of giving food to those who fear Him and goes on to praise Him for the extraordinary redemption of His people. Verses 6 and 9 suggest that this is a reference to the escape of God's people from slavery in Egypt. All of these actions flow from God's graciousness and compassion. The word for "graciousness" in Psalm 111:4 is also used in Psalm 145. Read Psalm 145:8-9. How is God described in verse 8?

gracious - compassionate
slow to anger - rich in Love

7-
As a result of His grace and compassion, what comes in verse 9?

for all He has made

7-10-
Read Psalm 136. These words are a reminder for us to be thankful for God's graciousness. What are some of the reasons this psalm gives for praising God for His grace?

great wonder
understanding

The refrain "His love endures forever" is a reminder that God's graciousness knows no limits, and the repetition of the phrase "Give thanks" is a reminder for us to be thankful for His never-ending compassion.

Dear Lord, thank You for pouring out Your grace on me. Your steadfast love and kindness to me are wonderful. Amen.

7-27-17

REFLECTION AND APPLICATION

*Father, sustain me with Your abundant grace. Increase my knowledge of
how to live in grace. Thank You for sending Jesus, the source of grace. Amen.*

We all have anxieties and various difficult situations, but we can rely
on God's grace to help us face them. That's what Darlene did.

When Darlene's children were all under six years old, she faced many
sleepless nights. The children rotated waking so that a little one roused
her every hour. She never fell back to sleep easily and it seemed that as
soon as she nodded off, another babe would wake her. In the wee hours
of the morning, Darlene often begged God to let her have at least one
hour of sleep. Through several nearly sleepless nights, she prayed. But
God kept reminding her of 2 Corinthians 12:9: "My grace is sufficient
for you."

Darlene finally chose to pray that God's grace and time would be
sufficient. Shortly after she prayed, she fell asleep peacefully, trusting
God to provide enough sleep. When the next young one cried out, she
had only had 15 minutes of uninterrupted sleep—but she woke refreshed as though she had slept enough.

Since that time, Darlene gives each of her weaknesses and whatever
she lacks to God—and God always provides enough of whatever is
needed: sleep, patience, food, money or other blessings to meet the day's
problems.

Many of us face situations just as frustrating as Darlene's. Yet we, like
her, can learn that God's grace is sufficient for every circumstance.
What situations are you facing right now that are causing you worry?

Marvin's illness

the weakness in my legs & back

Review Philippians 4:4-6. What can you rejoice in right now regarding the problem?

1 maybe they have an opportunity for a new career study.

2 when I do my therapy I seem to be going strength

The verses also remind us to respond gently. Consider the people involved in your problem. How can you show gentleness to them?

by prayer

Philippians 4:6 is a reminder to dwell on truth and good thoughts. Read Philippians 4:8. What good thoughts can you think about today?

1 I praise for the Drs in all the places they are taking Mason.

2. was so happy to see Hunter & he in enjoying swimming pool.

The end of verse 6 is a reminder to present your needs to God with thanksgiving. As you pray for grace for your situation, be thankful that God listens and responds to your needs.

Gracious Father, I trust You to provide enough grace for today. Continue renewing my mind that I might praise You and give You my worries. Amen.

8-8-11

REFLECTION AND APPLICATION

Day 7

Father, You are gracious to reach out and fill me with enough grace for today. Let Your strength show in my weakness. Amen.

John Bradford, an English reformer who was martyred in 1555, gave up a good career as a paymaster to study the Bible. He left his job because it included fraud and cover-ups that he no longer could take part in, and instead became a preacher. Under the reign of Queen Mary I, sometimes called "Bloody Mary," John was arrested on a false charge of inciting a riot.

From his prison in the Tower of London, John watched unknown criminals being led to execution and uttered the words, "There goes John Bradford, but for the grace of God!" He believed that only God's grace had kept him from a life of corruption.

John spent the rest of his life in prison, not complaining, but studying God's Word and writing about it, especially about grace. Part of the time he shared a cell with three other reformers who encouraged one another. When led to his own execution, John publicly forgave those who wronged him and encouraged another man sentenced to die, "Be of good comfort, brother, for we shall have a merry supper with the Lord this night!"[1]

Grace changes our hearts and our thinking so that we have freedom in spite of our circumstances or surroundings. Prison cannot separate us from God's grace or love.

Review Titus 2:11-15. What is our real hope, which helps us focus on God and not on our situation?

the grace of God

How have you been changed by God's grace?

I think I'm a more forgiving person
I can see my own falls

Compassion helps us support one another as we walk together on our journey. John Bradford had fellowship in prison. Paul felt connected to other Christians while in prison and that encouraged him. God has brought you to First Place 4 Health to give you encouragement and help. How have you been encouraged by members of your group?

_____

_____

_____

_____

How can you encourage others in your group?

_____

_____

_____

_____

How is God's grace guiding you to make better choices to live an upright life?

_____

_____

_____

_____

Paul began and ended most of his letters with thoughts on grace. John Bradford wrote letters to encourage others. Start a grace journal to record how God gives you grace each day, and consider sharing it with a friend.

Father, thank You for grace for each day and for the support of others You have brought into my life. Help me be encouraged and to encourage the members of my group. Amen.

Note
1. "Life of Master John Bradford: Some Account of the Rev. John Bradford, Prebendary of St. Paul's, and Martyr, a.d. 1555," Internet Christian Library. http://www.icl net.org/pub/resources/text/ipb-e/epl-10/web/bradford_life.html.

Group Prayer Requests

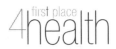

Today's Date: _____

Name	Request

Results

_____

_____

_____

_____

_____

grace to be
ourselves

SCRIPTURE MEMORY VERSE

For you created my inmost being; you knit me together in my mother's womb. I praise you because I am fearfully and wonderfully made; your works are wonderful, I know that full well.

PSALM 139:13-14

Perhaps you are knitting a sweater as you await a grandchild's birth. You have not seen his face, but you know he is a boy. You knit each stitch and pray for your grandson. You already love him and know that he will be a delight to his parents.

His brother and sister are also preparing for his birth by sorting toys for him, preparing a place for him to sleep and discussing names. But God is doing much more to prepare. He is creating this little boy and knitting his cells together in the womb. He has plans and a purpose for this little life.

God also created you, carefully knitting every cell together in your body. He had a plan for your life and counted the days before they began. He loved you before your mother knew you existed. He poured out His grace on you even when you remained hidden from the world in your mother's womb. God wants you to like yourself because He took the time to create you, but His plan did not end with creating you. Life began at that time and so did His desire for you to grow in grace and knowledge.

This week you will discover how much God loves you. You can love and accept yourself because you are wonderfully made. He chose to create you and made plans for your life before you were born. God's plan brought you to First Place 4 Health to restore your balance and health.

You can change and accept the plans God has for you to be healthy and full of wonderful works that show His grace to the world.

Day 1 — CREATED WITH GRACE

Gracious Father, You have a purpose for me with plans to prosper me. Give me grace to follow those plans. Amen.

Since Eve exclaimed that God had given her a son, people have marveled at the wonder of a newborn baby. The evidence of design and intricate wholeness of an infant shows God's grace. You are not a mistake, but a person God made with love.

Read Genesis 4:1 and 33:5. How did these parents describe their children?

God sent
with the help of God

Jacob's birth was a direct result of his father Isaac's prayer to open his wife's womb. Isaac, son of Abraham, was a promised child from God. (You can read more about these births in Genesis 25:21 and Genesis 17:16-18; 18:10-18; 21:1-3.) From the beginning, God's people recognized that each child is a gift of grace. Read Psalm 139:13-16. How did God make you?

He knit me together in my mother's womb

Look up Jeremiah 29:11-14. What plans does God have for your life?

future & hope

7-10-11

When He created you, God understood that you might be captivated by the world and enslaved to pleasures and poor choices. That is why He made a way to restore you. If you seek Him, He will bring you back from any captivity. He has a purpose for your life and gave you gifts and talents to help you fulfill that purpose. What are some thoughts people expressed to you in your childhood about talents they noticed? These are part of what God will use to accomplish His will for your life.

According to Matthew 10:29-30, how detailed is God's knowledge of you?

Every thing before I was ever born.

Read John 10:10. Jesus came to give you what kind of life? What does that mean to you?

full life

Turn to Proverbs 3:5-6. What can help you discover God's plans and how can you let Him direct you?

trust and acknowledge the Lord

Acknowledging God and trusting in Him means putting God first. That's the heart of First Place 4 Health. Putting God first helps everything else fall into place. Looking to God's ways directs you to the right decisions, in big and small life choices. How is acknowledging God helping you make healthier choices?

Take a walk today and notice all God created around you. Thank Him for His creations. Then at home, look in a mirror and thank God for creating you.

Creator Father, thank You for creating me and loving me. You know me intimately, including my weaknesses. As I commit my way to You, give me strength to follow Your direction for my life. Amen.

8-24-17   8-31-17

9-26-17

Day 2

GROWING IN GRACE

Dear Lord, I am thankful that You chose to make me and guide my growth. Help me grow in grace. Amen.

Many people enjoy gardening: watching the seeds spring up, grow and blossom. With all the children God creates, He continues to lavish love and grace upon each new life. Let's look at the growth process and learn how we can also grow in grace, starting with a look at Jesus growing up.

Read Luke 2:40 and 2:52. What happened as Jesus grew?

he was filled with wisdom
he had the graces of God upon him

According to 2 Peter 3:18, how are we to grow?

grow in the grace and knowledge of our
Lord

We are urged to increase in grace and knowledge of Jesus. Knowledge and grace are connected; when combined, they produce wisdom within us as we grow. As we apply ourselves to acquire knowledge, God showers us with grace to help us put that knowledge into practice, which leads to growth. First Place 4 Health is designed to help you grow in each area of your life—spiritual, mental, emotional and physical. In what ways are you growing in each of these areas? Be specific. Then rate your growth on a scale from 1 to 10. Put a star by the weakest area and make a commitment to gain knowledge and grow in grace this week.

Spiritual

studying my bible study more often

| 1 | 2 | 3 | 4 | 5 | 6 | 7 | 8 | 9 | 10 |

Mental

I am learning to stay focused on my goal

| 1 | 2 | 3 | 4 | 5 | 6 | 7 | 8 | 9 | 10 |

Emotional

I try to be happy & have a positive attitude

| 1 | 2 | 3 | 4 | 5 | 6 | 7 | 8 | 9 | 10 |

Physical

I am doing more exercising

| 1 | 2 | 3 | 4 | 5 | 6 | 7 | 8 | 9 | 10 |

9 - 14 - 11

Read 3 John 2-4. As John's friend Gaius walked in the truth, what was John's prayer for him? How might "walking in truth" bring this same blessing to you?

enjoy good health and all may go well

Look up Daniel 1:8-15. In this passage, the chief official was operating under worldly wisdom, but Daniel's wisdom came from God—and God honored Daniel's knowledge of healthy living by showing him grace. How will you grow in your knowledge of healthy living this week?

As we draw closer to God, He blesses us with more grace. As you study and live His Word, you will grow in knowledge of God and in His grace.

Father, thank You for Your grace and for helping me grow closer to You. Help me to understand Your Word. Amen.

Day 3

ACCEPTANCE

Father, thank You for loving me. Fill me with Your glorious grace and help me see myself through Your eyes and with Your love. Amen.

Many people suffer from low self-esteem and poor self-image. Those thoughts are not from God. You are His design. He created you. You are His work of art, and His love for you cannot be measured. Let's look at ourselves from God's perspective to understand how He created us with loving care.

Read Ephesians 1:2-6. How do these words tell you that God loves and accepts you?

_____

_____

_____

_____

Before He even created the world, God planned to create you. (And you thought waiting nine months for a baby's birth was a long time!) Just as a mother loves her child before he is born, God loved you long before you arrived. What word is used along with grace in Ephesians 1:2? How is God's love related?

_peace_____

_____

_____

Peace comes when we believe the truth about God's love for us—and belief is something we choose. We do not have to believe the lies we tell ourselves; we can choose to believe God's Word instead. Look up Jeremiah 31:3. How does God describe His love for you?

_everlasting love_____

_____

_____

_____

The word "drawn" in this verse is the Hebrew word *mashakh*, which means "draw, extend, develop." God created us and is developing us with His everlasting love and kindness! Because He has already accepted us, we must learn to accept ourselves and each other. According to Romans 15:7, what does acceptance do?

_bring praise to God_____welcome

_____

_____

10-5-17

How has your group shown that they accept you? How have you shown the other group members that you accept them?

We have become so close we share our trials as well as our joys

What is one thing you can do this week to let your loved ones know that they are accepted?

Tell them I love them and I'm praying for them

Turn to 1 Corinthians 15:10. What do the words "by the grace of God I am what I am" make you think about yourself? What has God's grace accomplished within you?

I hope I'm a better person

As you live in grace, you will continue to develop and accept yourself as the person God loves and created with care.

Father, thank You for accepting me and for creating me exactly as You envisioned. Help me grow in grace. Amen.

10-12

Day
4

GRACE AND WISDOM

Father, how wonderful is Your grace that fills me. Help me seek Your wisdom and not worldly wisdom to live a holy life that glorifies You. Amen.

You may not have a PhD in physics or even feel smarter than a fifth grader, but you can have something more valuable: godly wisdom. This is not the same as worldly wisdom. Godly wisdom looks beyond personal gain in the present to eternal blessings. Wisdom from God will help you live better now by making wiser choices, but those choices will be based on pleasing God, rather than yourself. The other wonderful thing about godly wisdom is that it is available to everyone, by God's grace.

Read 2 Corinthians 1:12. Why do you think Paul contrasted "the holiness and sincerity that are from God" with "worldly wisdom"? How are they different?

Our accomplishment are from God

According to this verse, grace helps a person make godly choices rather than worldly ones. The difference is God's wisdom. Turn to Proverbs 4:7-13. What are some benefits of wisdom?

God is leading us on the right
hold on to His instruction

What godly wisdom have you learned in First Place 4 Health?

Verse 9 describes wisdom placing a "garland [or wreath] of grace" on the head of those who value her. "Grace" in this phrase means kindness or favor. Can you think of someone you know who glows with kindness and radiates an inner beauty? Explain.

10-19-17

Read James 3:13-18. According to this verse, how are earthly and godly wisdom different?

unspiritual & from the devil
from heaven is pure, peace loving &
full of mercy

Read James 1:5-6. How do you get wisdom? What keeps you from receiving it?

if you ask for wisdom be ready to
receive it.
we have to believe

According to Psalm 19:7 and Psalm 111:10, what are the sources of godly wisdom?

The LORD
fear of the Lord brings understanding

The wisdom we receive when we ask, study God's Word and worship God is according to His grace—and it will be enough for each day.

> *Gracious Father, thank You for guiding me to First Place 4 Health. Give me the wisdom I need by Your grace. Amen.*

10-26-17

Day 5

RESTORATION

> *Dear Father, thank You for taking time and care to make me special. Help me follow the plans You have for me. Amen.*

God makes each person with great love and care. He also gives them free will to make choices, including the choice to disobey Him. The Bible calls this disobedience "sin." Our sins separate us from God. In order to draw close to Him, we must be restored. Our God-given free will allows us to make poor health choices, which can cause problems that include weight gain, heart disease and fatigue. But just as when we sin, God wants to restore us. Let's look at promises in Scripture that bring the hope of restoration.

Read 1 Peter 5:10. What does the God of all grace allow you to do for a little while? In what ways will He restore you?

suffer and then He will restore you

Look up Psalm 139:23-24. How might God's testing you start the process of restoration?

if I know I'm dont belong I'll try to do right, & God is with me

According to 1 John 1:8-9, who has sinned, and what will God do about it? How does forgiveness relate to restoration?

God will forgive our sins of we confess them.
We start of fresh & forgiven

11-2-17

Read Psalm 23:1-3. These verses describe the psalmist's vision of resting in God. What does rest, which is so important for healthy living, have to do with restoration?

rest restores all part of our body.
spiritual, emotional

11-16-17

According to Paul's words in Galatians 5:16-25, if we choose to walk by God's Holy Spirit, what fruit will grow in our lives? How are those qualities different from the sinful nature?

_____

_____

_____

Walking by the Spirit changes us from the inside out. We turn from selfish to selfless desires and become more gentle, self-controlled, loving and joyful. The Spirit will help us resist fleshly temptations. Yet as fruit on a tree takes time to grow, so, too, the fruits of the Spirit may take time to grow. You can do your part to nurture growth by praying and studying God's Word. Look up Psalm 51:10. Rewrite this verse in your own words, making it your prayer for restoration.

_____

_____

_____

_____

Gracious Father, restore me completely. Help me be steadfast in following You. Thank You, Lord. Amen.

Day
6

REFLECTION AND APPLICATION

God, You are the Potter, the one who forms us. Help us see the beauty You created in us. Amen.

One day, a woman went on a tour of a glass factory with her husband and her daughter. Her husband took her daughter to the showroom to shop. The daughter was fascinated by the swirling colors that emerged as the craftsmen blew the liquid glass and formed each piece into a unique, one-of-a-kind shape, and she wanted to help her dad choose a vase as a birthday gift for her mom.

Later, the daughter went up to her mother and anxiously said, "Daddy bought you a pretty present for your birthday, even though it has a few dents in it. The colors are pretty, Mom, so don't be upset when you open it." A few days later, the woman smiled when she unwrapped the gift: an exquisite vase with three carefully crafted indentations. It had taken gentle but firm pressure to create the "dents" without breaking the vase. Her daughter hadn't realized that making three matching indentations, which increased the artwork's value, took great skill.

The vase is a valuable treasure to those who understand the care and skill involved in its making. Like the daughter, we are sometimes tempted to see our "dents" as flaws until we see God's care and skill at work in our lives. We can learn to value the beauty of His handiwork. Instead of fretting over our inabilities and shortcomings, we can remember to focus on God, the Craftsman, who formed us.

Read Isaiah 64:8. List a few things you would like to change about yourself. Pray for God to show you the beauty He sees in you, His creation.

_____

_____

_____

Now list a few compliments you have recently received about your character or actions. How do these reflect how God is working in your life?

_____

_____

_____

This week we studied how God created us by His grace and how we are to grow in grace and knowledge. How is First Place 4 Health helping you grow in grace and knowledge?

_____

_____

_____

How do you most want to grow in the coming weeks?

_____

_____

_____

On slips of paper, write a compliment for each member of your group to give them this week to encourage their continuing growth in grace and knowledge.

Gracious Father, continue to mold and shape me. Help me to accept Your plan for me and to follow Your purpose for my life. Amen.

Day 7 — REFLECTION AND APPLICATION

Father, You made me and know me intimately. You also know the poor choices I have made. Yet You forgive my sins and You promise to restore me. Help me be steadfast and firm. Amen.

God offers us restoration, rest and wisdom. Adequate rest and healthy choices are important aspects of a balanced life, while godly wisdom guides us to make good choices that result in peace and produce good fruits.

Look back over the week's lessons. Pray over each promise of God for restoration. Which of these means the most to you right now on your journey toward health?

_____

_____

_____

Recite this week's memory verse as you look in a mirror. Thank God for your hair, eyes, face shape and all the features He designed for you. Ask Him to let you see the beauty He sees. Thank Him for the talents He gave you and ask Him to help you use them wisely.

Next, look at baby pictures of yourself and photos from the past years. Look at your smiles. Thank God for the joys you have experienced, and ask Him for restoration of past hurts. Ask Him to help transform your life to be more balanced and healthy.

Finally, consider how you are growing in grace and knowledge. How will you apply this growth in practical ways for your life? Consider steps you will take this week to rest and make good choices. Write down what you will resolve to do in each of the following areas to improve or maintain good health:

Rest

_____
_____
_____

Your relationship with God

_____
_____
_____

Forgiveness needed

_____
_____
_____

Wisdom desired

_____
_____
_____

Gracious Father, thank You for walking with me and giving
me grace for each day. Search me and restore me in every way.
Please continue to lead me in Your way. Amen.

Group Prayer Requests

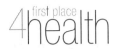

Today's Date: ___

Name	Request

Results

_____

_____

_____

_____

_____

_____

saved by grace

12-7-11

Blood is sometimes called the "river of life" because it transports nutrients and oxygen through the body to keep cells and organs healthy.

When the blood supply is cut off, muscles cramp and it becomes painful to move. This happens because the waste produced by the body's conversion of oxygen to energy, rather than being carried away by free-flowing blood, builds up within the muscles. Once the pressure is released, blood rushes back in to carry away those toxins and the pain is relieved.

Blood not only brings oxygen to the whole body; it also cleanses the body. T-cells within the blood release chemicals that kill invading organisms. B-cells become plasma when bacteria invades, producing antibodies to fight off infection. White blood cells, or leukocytes, help fight infection as well. Neutrophils remove cell debris and bacteria.[1]

Leviticus 17:11 says that the life of every creature is "in the blood"—and scientists and doctors have been proving this verse true with every new discovery they make of the blood's amazing abilities! This week, we will talk about the blood that cleanses us even more deeply than our miraculous human blood. The blood of Jesus, shed on the cross, is our very lifeline to heaven and eternity. And by God's grace, the blood of Jesus is freely available to everyone.

THE GRACIOUS HAND OF GOD

Father, I am thankful for how You graciously forgive me of my sins. Amen.

Blood clots prevent blood from flowing though the veins or arteries and can cause a stroke or other serious problems. Yet a clot is not immediately obvious—after all, it's in the veins and can't be seen from the outside! Only certain symptoms indicate a clot's presence. When a person has a blood clot, that person needs medical attention to break up or dissolve it to allow the blood to flow again.

Sin is like an unseen blood clot. It cuts off our life in God and can cause immense damage. Plus, it is undetectable until the Healer recognizes the symptoms and makes a diagnosis. God's forgiveness is what dissolves the clot. We can see a picture of this process in the book of Nehemiah. Nehemiah was a Jewish leader whose ancestors had been captured when the Babylonians took Jerusalem in 587 B.C. In 446 B.C., about 80 years after the Persians subdued the Babylonian Empire, Nehemiah lived in exile in Susa, which was the capital of the Persian Empire. The outward "symptom" we see in the book of Nehemiah is a broken city wall around Jerusalem, while the inner need to restore relationship with God is clearly present but not as obvious.

Today, we will look at how God dealt with the broken wall and relationships through His grace.

Read Nehemiah 1:3-7. When Nehemiah heard about the "symptom" of the broken wall, what did he do?

he wept & prayed

In Nehemiah's prayer, what did he confess?

Isralee confess sins
we have not obeyed your commands

After some months of prayer and fasting, the Persian king noticed Nehemiah's sadness. When he heard about the tragedy of its walls, he allowed Nehemiah to go to Jerusalem to see what he could do about it. In Nehemiah 2:8, to what did Nehemiah attribute the king's permission to provide supplies for the wall?

provide material to rebuild the wall

12-21-17 2:8, 98

When Nehemiah shared that the gracious hand of God was with him, how did the people respond (see verse 18)?

Lets start rebuilding

Read Nehemiah 6:15-16. How long did it take to rebuild the wall and what did the surrounding nations realize once it was rebuilt?

52 days
work was done with the help of God

In less than two months, the people rebuilt a wall that lay in ruins for 70 years. We find in Nehemiah 7 that, after the wall was rebuilt, the priests read the Book of the Law. As the people listened, they realized that they had turned away from God and sinned. According to Nehemiah 9:1-2, how did the people react?

stood and confess their sins

The people wanted to repent and be restored. In Nehemiah 9 we read of a public confession. The priests reminded the people how God had delivered their ancestors from slavery in Egypt. Then they all recounted their sins and recalled God's loving kindness and grace. Now turn to Nehemiah 9:31-33. What do the priests say about God's graciousness and His covenant with His people?

God acted faithfully to them while they still sinned

According to Nehemiah 10:28-29, what did the people agree to do?

to follow the Law of God

God restored the covenant with His people. He forgave their sins *and* gave them grace to repair the walls! When we repent of our sins, our gracious God forgives and restores us—both inside and out.

> *Dear Lord, thank You for forgiving me. Give me grace to live a godly life. Amen.*

2 - 15 - 18

Day 2 PLAN OF SALVATION

Gracious God, fill me with Your grace today. Help me comprehend all that You do for me. Amen.

Every three seconds, someone in America needs a blood transfusion.[2] Afterward, many recovering people feel as though they have received new life, a second chance to live and make better choices. But there's an even greater life-giving "blood transfusion": the sacrifice Christ made through His death on the cross. Today we'll study what it means to be saved by grace and the blood of Jesus.

Read Ephesians 1:7-8. What do we receive from the blood of Jesus?

redemption, forgiveness of sins lavished on us with all wisdom & understanding

What words describe the grace of God in these verses?

riches of Gods grace

Through God's grace, we receive forgiveness and redemption. Read 1 John 1:7-9. What do these verses tell us the blood of Jesus does?

the blood of Jesus purifies us from all sin

What do we need to do in order to be forgiven?

Confess our sins

According to Romans 5:5-7, why did Jesus want to die for each of us?

because we were all sinners

The deeper question is why God would *want* to offer us this gift. Turn to John 3:16. Why did God offer His Son, Jesus, the greatest gift we could ever receive?

because He loved us & we could have eternal life.

Read Acts 2:21 and Romans 10:9, which tell us how we can receive God's gracious gift of salvation. What do we need to do?

you have to believe & call on God

If you have not yet told God that you believe in His Son, that you are sorry for your sins and then called on Him to be Lord of your life, stop and do so now. You don't need fancy words. He loves you and just wants you to call on Him. You can start by praying the prayer below:

Dear God, thank You for sending Your Son to die for me. I am truly sorry for my sins and ask Your forgiveness. I believe that Jesus died, shed His blood for me and rose from the grave. Save me by Your grace. Amen.

2-22-18

Day 3

AMAZING GRACE

Dear Lord, I rejoice that You saved me and forgave my sins. I am thankful that You gave Your blood for me. I rejoice in my salvation. Amen.

It is amazing that God would reach out to us and give us the gift of eternal life! Many people have marveled in the wonder of God's grace of salvation and expressed their thoughts in song. One such individual was John Newton, who around 1772 penned these lines in what would become the popular hymn "Amazing Grace":

Amazing grace, how sweet the sound
That saved a wretch like me!
I once was lost but now am found
Was blind but now I see.[3]

Read 1 Timothy 1:14-17. How did Paul consider himself?

_____

_____

_____

Paul was saved by God's grace, but that didn't keep him free of trouble. His life, as recorded in the book of Acts, was filled with persecution, imprisonment, shipwrecks and beatings. Grace did not always take John

Newton out of trouble, either, but it always sustained both Paul and Newton through hard times. What dangers or snares have you come through with God's grace?

_____

_____

_____

_____

4.

Turn to Acts 16:22-34, which recounts an incredible story of God's grace through the lives of Paul and Silas. What question did the jailer ask about salvation, and what answer did he receive?

_____

_____

_____

4-12-18

Read Isaiah 12:2-6. Besides singing for joy, what do these verses (especially verse 4) suggest we should do in response to God's salvation?

_____

_____

_____

How did you feel when you were first saved, and how have you shared your joy?

_____

_____

_____

_____

What are a few of your favorite songs that help you to celebrate your salvation? Find some time to sing them today!

Dear Lord, You are so gracious to forgive me and bring me through troubles. Thank You for Your grace and for the gift of salvation. Amen.

6 - 14

CALLED TO A HOLY LIFE OF GRACE

Lord, thank You for saving me. Show me how to live as a believer. Amen.

It's wonderful to be saved, but it is just the beginning of being a Christian and getting to know Jesus. The lives of the early Christians, recorded in the book of Acts, show us what's next and how we should live once we have been saved. Today we'll look at the Early Church at Antioch, where the worldwide mission of the church began. We'll discover what God desires of us once we have accepted His gift of salvation.

Read Acts 11:19-23. How did people in Antioch learn about Jesus? According to verse 21, what helped the men from Cyprus and Cyrene tell them the good news?

the Lords hand was with them

When the church at Antioch began, what did Barnabas discover and encourage the believers to do?

believe in the grace of God and encourage people to remain loyal to the Lord

What did people see in Barnabas?

the grace of God

6-21-18

Barnabas means "son of encouragement." He is first mentioned in Acts 4:36-37. His real name was Joseph, but people called him Barnabas because of his great gift of encouragement. Barnabas saw evidence of God's grace and encouraged others in their faith. In Acts 11:25-30, Barnabas brought Paul (then called Saul) to Antioch. What did Paul and Barnabas do for a year?

met with the church & taught
disciples where first called Christians
in Antioch.
6-28

These verses show us the next steps for new believers. They studied their faith, met together and shared their resources. And as they did, God added to their numbers. God wants us to follow their example—these people who followed Christ so passionately that people labeled them "Christians." Turn to Ephesians 2:8-10. What did God plan when He created you?

7-19-18

The good works God planned for you are not a means to salvation, for we know that salvation is a gift. Rather, our good works are how we team up with Him. In Antioch, the Christians heard about a need and re-sponded—they did the good works God had planned in advance for them to do. Barnabas is another example of how a Christian identified and used his gift to do good works. Read 2 Timothy 1:6-9. Why have we been saved (see verse 9)?

God called us to a Holy Life because
of his own purpose & grace.

The phrase "called to a holy life" is used as a reminder that God's purpose for you is sacred and meaningful. It flows from His grace. According to Ephesians 4:1-3, how can a Christian live a life worthy of his or her calling?

be completely humble & gentle, bearing
with one another in love

As you continue living your holy calling to do good works, allow God's grace to shape you into a Christian in the model of the earliest believers: humble, gentle, patient, loving and unified in the power of the Spirit!

Dear Lord, show me Your purpose for my life and help me to respond with love and holiness. Amen.

8-2-18   8-9-18

Day 5 — GRACE AND ETERNAL LIFE

Dear Lord, thank You for the gift of eternal life and for the joy of being with You forever. Amen.

The life of a baby in the womb is much different than its life out of the womb. In the small, dark place, a baby is sustained by the umbilical cord, through which blood flows from its mother to sustain and nurture it for the life the baby is meant to live after birth. The world into which the baby is born is full of sights, sounds, people and love that it could never imagine or comprehend until after delivery.

In a similar way, we cannot comprehend the life we will live in the place God is preparing for us for all eternity. It will be a place of sights, sounds, people and everlasting love that we can only begin to imagine here in our dark "womb." Until then, however, we are sustained and nurtured by the flow of Christ's blood, which prepares us for an eternity with Him.

Read John 14:1-2. What did Jesus say about heaven?

There are many rooms.

8-23-18

In Matthew 8:10-11, what glimpse of heaven does Jesus give us through these words? What does this mean to you?

8-23-18

Now turn to Revelation 4:2-11. This passage gives us another glimpse of heaven, described in words that may be difficult to understand. There's a good reason for that: Heaven is hard to describe in human words! What do you think the author of Revelation wants us to know about heaven from his description?

Beautiful, breathtaking, glorious all praising God. Holy, Holy, holy

8-30-18

These promises give us a peek at our future, which can bring us hope for our present. Let's look at how eternal life impacts present living. Read Romans 5:20-21. When grace reigns in our lives, what happens?

brings eternal life
takes away grief

According to 2 Thessalonians 2:14-17, what will sustain us when we are tempted to fall?

by grace God gave of eternal encouragement

Sin still exists in this world, but the hope of eternal life changes how we view problems. We can see they will pass and we can look forward to something better. This confidence helps us stand firm with expectant joy.

Joy is not the same thing as happiness. Our word "happiness" is derived from the Latin root *hap*—the word "haphazard" shares the same root. Happiness is a temporary reaction to fleeting circumstances. Joy, on the other hand, is the response of the believer to good news, such as the shepherds' joy when they heard about the birth of Christ (see Luke 2:8-20). The word for "joy" in the New Testament is *chara*, meaning cheer, gladness or celebration, and its root word is *charis*, meaning grace. Joy is an attitude shaped by God's grace in our lives, not a reaction.

Read 1 Peter 1:3-9. What does verse 8 tell us about joy?

_____

_____

_____

Peter understood that believing even though we do not see is the difference between *sight* and *insight*. It is insight—a perspective brought by salvation through God's grace—that offers us joy in the midst of trying circumstances.

> *Lord, help me hold on to the hope of eternity in my heart that I may face pain and suffering with the joy of my salvation. Amen.*

9-16-18

Day 6

REFLECTION AND APPLICATION

Dear Father, by Your grace I am saved. Give me the grace to do the works You have planned for me. Amen.

In the Day Three study, we noted that John Newton is remembered for his famous song "Amazing Grace." The words reflect his change in life from a bitter slave trader to a Christian preacher. When he was 6, John's godly mother died, and at 11 he went to sea with his stern father. Several years later, after his father had retired, John was forced to work on a man-of-war ship under harsh conditions. He deserted the ship, was recaptured and then flogged. At his request, he was then exchanged to serve on a slave ship. John spent four years in the slave trade, eventually becoming captain of a slave ship.

During a fierce storm at sea, John concluded that only God's grace could save him, so he cried out for His mercy. He and the ship survived, but the experience changed his life. John Newton always considered that the true day of his conversion.

Several years after the storm, John left the slave trade and studied under evangelist George Whitfield. He had still traded slaves after becoming a Christian, but he took care to treat the slaves well. Yet as he grew in his faith, he knew that he could no longer buy and sell people created by God. He became an abolitionist, a preacher and a songwriter. Twenty years after his conversion, John Newton wrote "Amazing Grace." Looking back over his life, he saw how God's grace changed him, and he rejoiced.

John's tombstone reads, "John Newton, Clerk, once an infidel and libertine, a servant of slaves in Africa, was, by the rich mercy of our Lord and Saviour Jesus Christ, preserved, restored, pardoned, and appointed to preach the faith he had long labored to destroy."[4]

A great storm caused John Newton to seek God. What caused you to turn to God and seek His grace?

_____

_____

_____

Once he was saved, John didn't change immediately. He slowly grew in his faith as he studied the Bible. Over time he committed himself to following God's direction and became a preacher. How have you changed since becoming a Christian? How does studying the Bible help in your growth?

_____

_____

_____

What changes do you want to make with God's grace?

_____

_____

_____

Has God been directing you to make changes in your life or called you to a ministry? In what way?

_____

_____

_____

*God, Your grace is amazing. Thank You for giving me grace so generously
every day. Amen.*

REFLECTION AND APPLICATION

Day
7

*Dear Lord, I want to follow You and live a holy life. Give me the grace to have
the patience, gentleness and love for others that You want me to develop. Amen.*

Christians in the Early Church at Antioch spent time learning their faith,
and then they practiced it. That's part of the calling to live a holy life of
grace. To stay accountable in your study, keep a journal to record what
you are learning, prayers answered and how God's grace is changing you.

On Day Four, we studied Ephesians 4:1-3. Those verses instruct us
to practice humility, gentleness, unselfishness, patience and love toward
one another and to work in a manner worthy of our calling. Reflect on
how you are doing in those areas and how you can improve. Take some
time today to journal about your progress.

When has the gentleness of someone impressed you? How?

_____

_____

_____

To whom do you need to be gentle? How can you do this?

_____

_____

_____

Have you observed someone acting unselfishly? In what ways has that
impressed you?

_____

_____

_____

How can you encourage others in the group to practice humility, gentleness, unselfishness, patience and love?

_____

_____

_____

Have you been impatient lately? If so, what can you do next time you encounter a similar situation?

_____

_____

_____

Some biblical scholars have suggested that the word "worthy" in Ephesians 4:1 can be understood both as "balanced" and "becoming." The implication is that, as we balance the knowledge of our calling with action, we become the people God created us to be. How are you learning to balance what you study with your actions?

_____

_____

_____

Dear Father, thank You for the gift of salvation. Help me to follow You more closely, to understand Your Word and to keep my hope fixed on You. Amen.

Notes

1. "White Blood Cell," Wikipedia.org, June 24, 2010. http://en.wikipedia.org/wiki/White_blood_cell.
2. "Someone Needs Blood Every 3 Seconds," Medicine.org, September 29, 2007. http://www.medicine.org/profiles/blogs/someone-needs-blood-every-3 (accessed May 2010).
3. John Newton, "Amazing Grace," first printed in Olney Hymns, 1779. It is believed that Newton first wrote the hymn as a poem to illustrate a sermon delivered on New Year's Day of 1773.
4. Al Rogers, "Amazing Grace: The Story of John Newton," July-August 1996. "http://www.anointedlinks.com/amazing_grace.html.

Group Prayer Requests

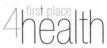

Today's Date: _9 - 13 - 18_

Name	Request
Jackson Church	
Hunter & Mason	
Ben King - toe	
Fish family	
Darla	

Results

_____

_____

_____

_____

_____

9-20-18

encouragement of grace

SCRIPTURE MEMORY VERSE
See to it, brothers, that none of you has a sinful, unbelieving heart that turns away from the living God. But encourage one another daily, as long as it is called Today, so that none of you may be hardened by sin's deceitfulness.
HEBREWS 3:12-13

It all started with anger.

In the coffee drive-thru, one driver was at first annoyed by the driver behind him, who honked and yelled at him to hurry up (as if he could make the line go any faster!). After his initial irritation, however, the first driver thought that the angry man might be having a bad day. Instead of retaliating in kind, he paid for the guy's coffee.

When the angry driver arrived at the window, he discovered that the man in front of him had already paid for his order! Lesson learned. The formerly angry driver paid for the next car's order to make amends for his bad behavior.

But it didn't stop there! The next driver, and the next, and the next all paid for the next customer's order . . . until more than 1,000 customers had done the same!

Kindness is contagious. It only takes one person to spark a chain-reaction that can touch the lives and hearts of thousands. This week, we will look at a parable about kindness, generosity and encouraging words to find out how gracious actions can impact people.

GRACE IN ACTION

Dear Lord, thank You for showing kindness and mercy to me.
Help me to be gracious today in passing on kindness to others. Amen.

"Good Samaritan laws" protect bystanders who come to the rescue of someone in need. The idea behind the laws is that no one should be penalized for seeing a need and trying to help, even if the situation turns out badly. If they could be sued for their attempts to save lives, there would probably be a lot fewer heroes!

Good Samaritan laws get their nickname from a story Jesus told about what it means to be a neighbor. Today we'll look at the Parable of the Good Samaritan to find out how we can put grace into action by showing mercy to someone in need.

Read 1 Thessalonians 5:11. What does "build each other up" mean to you? How does your First Place 4 Health group build each other up?

_____

_____

_____

Encouragement is a free gift we give to others, and we most often encourage those who are close to us. Yet Jesus wants us to look beyond people we know to anyone in need and to call them our neighbors. Let's examine the story Jesus shared about what it means to be a neighbor. Turn to Luke 10:25-37. What did the expert in the law know in his head about following God?

_____

_____

_____

9-27-15

First-century Jews tended to look down on Samaritans because of their mixed race. Most scholars agree that even though Jesus identified him only as "a man," the robbery victim was a Jew. The first two passersby were also Jews, yet they did not stop to help. What moved the Samaritan to help him (see verse 33)?

he took pity on him

How did the Samaritan show extravagant generosity?

he bandaged his wounds & took him to the inn & gave him money.

When have you received extraordinary generosity from someone? How did it feel?

Think about a few people beyond your circle of friends. Who is in need of a neighbor? How will you help him or her this week?

Time is limited and days are filled with busyness, but the Second Great Commandment isn't just a suggestion! "Loving your neighbor" is an essential part of our response to God's abundant grace. Build in time cushions of extra minutes in each day to allow time to respond to unexpected needs of others.

Dear Lord, thank You for always taking time to hear my prayers and respond to my needs. Help me be generous toward others. Amen.

10 - 4 - 18

RANDOM ACTS OF GRACE

Dear Father, let me be prepared when You delegate a task to me. Thank You for trusting me with the important job of showing grace to others. Amen.

The only time the word "innkeeper" is used in the New Testament is in the story of the Good Samaritan. While it may seem at first glance that the innkeeper is a background character in the parable, there are still things we can learn from him. After all, we sometimes find ourselves "in the background" of situations where there is a need. Read Luke 10:34-35. What responsibility did the innkeeper take on?

_____

_____

_____

_____

Caring for the robbery victim involved much more than giving him keys to a room and sending up room service three times a day—the man had been badly beaten and needed medical attention! And while the Samaritan gave him a few coins for expenses, the innkeeper had to take it on trust that he would be paid if the man's condition demanded more than what the money would cover. If the coins ran out, he would be faced with a choice: respond with compassion, as the Samaritan did, or make profit the bottom line. Have you ever been "delegated" to show mercy to someone? If so, how did you deal with that situation?

_____

_____

_____

When has someone enlisted you to help in a ministry?

_____

_____

_____

_____

In Matthew 25:34-40, what does God promise to those who help someone in need?

_____

_____

_____

It is important to give money to our church and to other organizations that are meeting the needs of hurting people, but it's clear from the Samaritan's and the innkeeper's example that it is also important to get personally involved. Why do you think Jesus makes such a big deal about getting up close and personal with those who are hurting?

_____

_____

_____

Think about the ministries your church has to your community's needs. What is one way you can get personally involved?

_____

_____

_____

What is the hardest part about getting involved? Are you insecure? Anxious that you won't have all the answers? Afraid you don't have enough time? Spend a few minutes evaluating your concerns, then write a short prayer asking God to open the right doors for you to show mercy.

_____

_____

_____

_____

_____

Lord, thank You for giving me the example of the innkeeper. Help me to accept the work You delegate and use it as an opportunity to encourage others.

10-25-

GRACIOUS WORDS

Dear Lord, I am encouraged by Your Word. Help me to encourage others today. Amen.

Words begin in our heart with our emotions. When a person is angry or upset, they may hide it in their expression but often the words spoken reveal their heart's condition. Likewise, when the heart is filled with love and grace, kindness flows in the speech. Turn to Matthew 12:34. What connection did Jesus make between the heart and speech?

if you have something in your heart
It will come out of your mouth

Now read Colossians 4:2-6. How would you describe speech that is "full of grace, seasoned with salt"?

mouth control - be happy

How do you think Paul's instructions in verses 2 to 5 relate to the command in verse 6 to speak with grace? What do praying, proclaiming Christ, being wise in relationships and making the most of every opportunity have to do with our heart's condition?

Happy Heart - be Joyfull

11-1-18

Let's look at the use of salt in the Bible to understand Colossians 4:6. In Leviticus 2:13, what were the ancient Israelites commanded to do with salt?

Salt is a preservative as well as a seasoning. In ancient times, salt provided the main means to preserve food, which made it valuable to people who did not have modern refrigeration. How do you think the preservative qualities of salt might represent God's enduring covenant with His people?

_____

_____

_____

Read Ephesians 4:29-32. How might these instructions help you to season your words with grace?

if we stop & think before we speak

_____

_____

Notice in this passage that Paul is talking about attitudes within our hearts, which lead to either words of grace or unwholesome words (verse 29). Think about a time when you said something unkind. Was the root of those words of bitterness, rage, rivalry, slander or malice? How might compassion and forgiveness have changed the outcome?

_____

_____

_____

_____

When forgiveness, kindness and compassion fill our hearts, what we say will reflect those positive feelings. When you hear yourself speaking angry words or unkind criticism, stop and do a heart check. Figure out what emotions triggered the outburst and ask forgiveness for the source of the negative attitudes.

Dear Lord, help my heart be full of gratitude and kindness. Let my speech be seasoned with salt and show me who needs encouragement today. Amen.

18 . 18
11-18

Day
4

TEAM SPIRIT

Dear Lord, thank You for giving me supportive friends. Help us work together through Your grace for Your glory. Amen.

God's grace saved Paul, who then spread encouragement and the good news everywhere he went. Paul met Priscilla and Aquila in Corinth, where they worked together as tentmakers. The couple became instructors in the Christian faith and traveled to Ephesus with Paul. In Ephesus, Aquila and Priscilla met Apollos, a Jewish believer, after Paul had left his friends to continue his missionary journeys (see Acts 18).

Paul sent greetings to the couple in his letter to the Romans, calling them his "fellow workers in Christ Jesus" (Acts 16:3). Even separated, Paul reached out to encourage his friends. Today we'll discover more about Priscilla, Aquila and Apollos and how they worked together to share their faith and to encourage one another. And we'll discover how grace is a common connection for team spirit.

Read Acts 18:24-27. What did Apollos not know about Jesus when he met Priscilla and Aquila?

He knew only about the baptism of John

What did Priscilla and Aquila do to help Apollos gain more understanding of the Lord?

they taught him the way of God

Hospitality builds friendship and trust, while words of encouragement and instruction shared in private are marks of a good coach or mentor. Away from public embarrassment, Apollos could listen and learn in the comfort of the home of his new friends. What did Apollos's new friends do to make sure he was also welcomed in Achaia?

_____

_____

_____

What happened once Apollos arrived in Achaia (see verse 27)?

_____

_____

_____

It may be that Priscilla, Aquila and the other believers in Ephesus learned their humble generosity from Paul, who emphasized it again and again. Paul believed that fellow workers in Christ should not take credit for themselves but do everything to help each other for God's glory. Read 1 Corinthians 3:3-10. How did Paul and Apollos work together for God's glory?

_____

_____

_____

In your own words, describe the Christian teamwork you see in verses 6 to 9. Who deserves the credit for the result?

_____

_____

_____

_____

Jealousy and strife should not be part of the Christian life. Encouraging one another keeps us focused on team spirit and helps us appreciate each individual's gifts and contributions. Today, think of some way that you are helping to be a "team player," especially in your First Place 4 Health group.

Lord, thank You for the community of Christian believers. Help me to appreciate each believer and do my part for the good of the team. Amen.

12-6-18

FRUITFUL WORDS

Dear Lord, let my words be pleasing to You and effective in encouraging others. Amen.

Our goal in speaking is to communicate—not just to emit sounds. The goal of communication is to connect with others and nurture relationships. The words we choose will either help or hinder this goal. Where they help, we can call these words "fruitful"; they bear the fruit of closer relationships, personal and spiritual growth, and positive change. Today we'll look at practical ways we can speak words that bear the fruit of communication.

Read Proverbs 18:20-21 and then rewrite these verses in your own words.

_____

_____

_____

God gives us food to help us grow. How can words be like good, satisfying food?

It fills us up with joy

_____

_____

Discouraging words and abusive language can dash a person's hopes and self-respect, while constructive words can bring life to a dream and encourage someone to improve and change. In order for our words to bear these encouraging fruits, we need to choose them carefully. Hebrews 13:15-16 talks about the fruit Christians should want to produce and how to nurture that fruit. According to this passage, what fruit should we bear with our lips?

Confess His name & praise

_____

_____

How are these two verses related? How does doing good to others proclaim your allegiance to Christ's name?

Christ always did good so should we

12 - 13 - 18

When the ancient Israelites presented a grain offering to God, it was to be offered without yeast or leavening (see Leviticus 2). Yeast was a symbol of sin, so the absence of it represented the worshiper's desire to be blameless before God. Look up 1 Corinthians 5:6-8. In these verses, believers are compared to two different batches of dough: one made with yeast and one made without. How are the two batches different? What does the yeast symbolize (see verse 8)?

The grain offering of the Old Testament was a symbol of the Israelites' thankfulness to God for His gracious provision. They offered the "firstfruits" of the harvest as thanks. In the metaphor of 1 Corinthians 5, God's grace through Christ's sacrifice has yielded another kind of harvest: us! What is one specific way you can offer the fruit of your words to Him in thanks?

Dear Lord, thank You for helping me bear fruit, which helps me share
Your grace with others. Help me to speak fruitful words. Amen.

REFLECTION AND APPLICATION

Dear Lord, help me to use words pleasing to You. Season my words with salt and anoint my lips with grace. Amen.

Jim traveled constantly for work, which made it difficult for him to stay connected with others and encourage them—until he remembered the letters Paul wrote to encourage his friends and other believers. Jim decided to send postcards to people from each place he stayed. He wrote little notes to encourage his pastor, his friends, the sick in his church and his family. He took time to find cards with photos that might interest each person.

Over time, people commented on how much Jim's notes meant to them. One lady who was bedridden in long-term care said that she felt as though she was traveling with him. His pastor mentioned that Jim's cards lifted his spirit and often came on days when he faced a church member's death or another crisis.

After the staff at one hotel noticed that Jim always asked for stamps and bought postcards when he stayed with them, they surprised him by setting up a mailing station where he could purchase the cards and stamps and write out his messages in one place.

Words don't always have to be spoken; in fact, written encouragements sometimes outlast verbalized words because they can be read again and again. Handwritten notes, email and online social networking sites give us an opportunity to encourage others in various ways.

Have you kept special notes, cards or emails from others? What about them is meaningful to you? How do they continue to encourage you?

Think of a few people with whom you don't interact on a regular basis. What are some ways you can get in touch to encourage them?

_____

_____

_____

_____

Jim's note-writing got a lot easier after the hotel staff helped him by setting aside a special place with everything he needed. Likewise, it's easier to stay on top of keeping in touch if we have a plan. Think about the people you would like to regularly encourage, and then come up with a simple plan. When will you do it? What supplies do you need?

_____

_____

_____

_____

Pastors and other leaders need extra encouragement. Take a few minutes today to write a kind note to your pastor, First Place 4 Health leader or other leader in your life—he or she needs to know how much their commitment and faithfulness means to you!

Dear Father, thank You for the encouragement of Your written Word.
Help me to encourage those around me. Amen.

REFLECTION AND APPLICATION

Day 7

Dear Father, help me influence others to be encouragers. Amen.

Military ships are not known as places of wholesome words. ("He swears like a sailor" is not just an empty cliché.) One sailor, tired of the constant foul language, asked to be transferred.

The sailor's commanding officer called him in to discuss his reasons for the change-of-duty request, and the young man explained that he just couldn't take any more cursing, insults and mean-spirited words. Rather than granting the sailor's request, the C.O. worked with the other officers to clean up the language and bad attitudes in the men's quarters. The result was great for everyone, even those men who had to learn to curb their tongues: friendly working relationships, peaceful living quarters and a team that respected each other.

Positive words can change bad attitudes and poor habits. Encouragement unites us with Christ, and then with other believers (see Philippians 2:1-2). Sharing love and a purpose draws us together. Today, let's look at how we use words and the changes we can make to share God's grace with others.

What is your normal morning greeting to those at home and at work?

Mornings are not always easy after a bad night's sleep or too little rest, but with God's grace we can wake with encouragement on our lips. Starting the day with prayer and Bible study may be helpful, too. What can you do to improve your greeting?

How do you usually react when you are angry?

How could a quick prayer help you season your reaction with grace?

_____

_____

_____

_____

_____

_____

Consider the person with whom you interact each day who is the hardest for you to encourage. What kind word will you say to him or her today? Plan ahead!

_____

_____

_____

_____

_____

Consider where you spend most of your time. At home? At work? How might a positive change in your words affect the whole atmosphere?

_____

_____

_____

_____

_____

For the next week, set aside time each night to evaluate your words. Review your interactions with people throughout the day and journal about where you spoke with kindness, where you can improve and what you will do differently the next day.

Dear Father, help me be an encourager. Let my words be
seasoned with grace. Thank You, Lord. Amen.

Group Prayer Requests

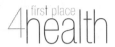

Today's Date: _____

Name	Request

Results

_____
_____
_____
_____
_____

Week Six

transformed by grace

SCRIPTURE MEMORY VERSE

*This righteousness from God comes through faith in Jesus Christ to all who believe.
There is no difference, for all have sinned and fall short of the glory of God, and are
justified freely by his grace through the redemption that came by Christ Jesus.*
ROMANS 3:22-24

When we feel thirsty, we know what to do. Our bodies let us feel the need for water, and we reach for a refreshing drink.

Scientific studies show that water is the best choice to relieve our thirst. Water lubricates the salivary juices so that we can swallow. It transports nutrients through the body and lubricates around tissues to absorb shock, especially protecting the brain, eyes, and spinal cord. Water also regulates body temperature by storing heat in the body and using evaporation of sweat for cooling.

Water is necessary for life. Without it, a person dehydrates. Signs of dehydration include dry mouth, warm skin, sleepiness, cramps, headaches and dizziness. Severe dehydration can cause fainting, heart failure, convulsions and even death.[1]

We need water daily and can get it from various sources. All fluids contain water, as do many foods. Some vegetables and fruits, such as celery and lettuce, are 90 percent water. Even many grain products are composed of one-third water.[2]

Thirst serves as the natural reminder that we need water. Alas, we don't have an internal system to remind us that we need grace or to motivate

LORD - God, Jesus, Spirit
Lord - God only

us to reach for the Source of grace. Yet we need it to live. Grace absorbs the shock of crisis, helps us to regulate our responses and emotions and saves us from sin. We need grace for eternal life. This week, we'll study how Jesus is our Source of grace.

Day 1

JESUS, THE SOURCE OF GRACE

Lord, I come to You, my Source of grace. Strengthen me for the work You want me to do. Amen.

Paul understood how grace had changed him and recognized the value of grace to other people's lives. He prayed for his friend Timothy to receive grace and advised him to be strong in the grace of Jesus. Paul's words to Timothy are valuable insights into the Source of grace.

Read 2 Timothy 1:1-2. What did Paul want for Timothy?

Grace, mercy, peace from God

What was the Source of grace Paul believed would strengthen Timothy?

God the Father & Christ Jesus our Lord.

Look up 2 Timothy 2:3-6. What metaphor did Paul use for being a Christian? How might this understanding help you to live a Christian life?

understand the Christian life and live the Christian life

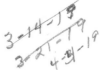

What two metaphors does Paul use in verses 5 and 6? How do these word pictures help you understand the grace you receive as you work for the Lord?

athlete - compete according to rules
farmer - 1st to receive share of crops

Soldiers, athletes and farmers discipline themselves to achieve their goals and expect results from their efforts. What are your goals for your Christian life? What results do you expect?

What are two actions you can take to pursue faith, love and peace?

It's unnatural to respond to hurtful words or actions with kindness, but with Christ's grace, it can be done. Rejoice that Jesus has given you grace for today.

Thank You, Lord, for giving me grace today. Help me to be kind and gentle to others that it might bring people to follow You. Amen.

LAVISH GRACE OF CHRIST

Day 2

Dear Lord, thank You for Your grace, a lavish gift that I don't deserve. Amen.

Christ's grace makes us strong and provides us with all we need. During His earthly ministry, Jesus noticed people's needs and reached out generously to help. Read Matthew 15:32-38. What did Jesus feel for the people? Why?

_____
_____
_____
_____

How did Jesus respond to their hunger?

_____
_____
_____
_____

How does the abundant supply of food illustrate God's endless and lavish supply of grace?

_____
_____
_____
_____

What has God done in your life that shows His lavish grace?

_____
_____
_____
_____
_____

Look up John 6:35,40. More than temporary food, what does Jesus want to give us? *The bread of life – the bread that is living*

Now turn to Titus 3:4-7. How did Jesus show mercy? What happens once we are justified by His grace?

hope of eternal life
we become heirs

The people who followed Jesus on that day long ago did nothing to earn the food He gave them through a miracle. Likewise, we have done nothing to earn eternal life or to be freed from the penalty of our sins. He has such great love and grace that He lavishes us with His saving grace, just as He met the needs of those hungry people and had so much left over. Jesus, the Source of grace, is an extravagant Giver. He gives because He loves us.

Dear Lord, thank You for Your compassion, for walking beside me and for understanding my needs. Give me the grace that I need. Amen.

RECEIVING GRACE

Day 3

Dear Lord, You give grace abundantly, without limit. Thank You for strengthening me. Amen.

Even as He suffered unimaginable agony on the cross, Jesus was ready to give grace. Read Luke 23:39-43. What took place between Jesus and the repentant criminal who hung beside Him?

One criminal insulted Jesus
one rebuked the other criminal

Jesus showed grace to the criminal

What did the criminal admit about the difference in himself and Jesus?

criminal was guilty & Jesus was not

5—16—19
6—13 = 9:00

Jesus' response to the criminal reveals how much He is ready to respond to anyone who turns to Him. The criminal made no reply to Jesus' astonishing promise; it's easy to believe that he was left speechless by such a lavish present. If we stop and consider Christ's grace, we should be awestruck with wonder, too. According to Ephesians 4:7, by what measure is grace given to us? Given what you have learned about Jesus' generosity, what does that mean?

_____

_____

_____

_____

Jesus is the Source of grace not only for our salvation but also for our growth with other believers. For that purpose, He gives us spiritual gifts by His grace. These gifts are not all the same, but they share a common goal: to connect us with Christ and to each other. Read Ephesians 4:11-16. What are the gifts listed in verse 11? Who are a few people you know who have been given these gifts?

_____

_____

_____

_____

What is the purpose of the various gifts (see verses 12-13)?

_____

_____

_____

_____

Just as a baseball team won't win very many games if every player is a pitcher, so too a team of Christians cannot accomplish God's purpose for them if they each have the same gifts. In accepting your gift and using it to build up the Body of Christ, God uses you to give His grace to others.

Your gifts are not for your glory but for His. According to 2 Corinthians 4:13-15, what happens as God's grace reaches more and more people?

_____

_____

_____

_____

God's grace is too much to keep to ourselves! The gifts He generously bestows help us to reach others with His grace, who in turn reach others. Are you amazed yet?

> *Dear Lord, thank You for dying that I might live. Help me share*
> *Your grace and gifts with others. Amen.*

6-20-19

ABOUNDING GRACE Day 4

Lord, help Your grace to flow through me to touch the hearts of others. Amen.

A farmer sows seeds, nurtures the crop and reaps a harvest. There's a correlation between the sowing and reaping. In a similar way, there is a correlation between the seeds we sow and the harvest we reap. Christ desires us to sow generosity and reap a harvest of abundant grace.

We respond best to God's grace by following His example. He gives generously, and as we follow His example He prospers our efforts with even more generosity and blessing. Today we will examine the relationship between sowing generosity and reaping an abundance of grace.

Read 2 Corinthians 9:6-11. What kind of harvest does God promise if we sow generously?

result in thanksgiving to God.

_____

_____

8-1-7ᵃ

According to verse 11, what will happen when God enlarges the "harvest of your righteousness"?

We will be made rich in every way.

8-8-19

By His grace, what does God provide so that you can sow generously (see verse 8)?

have all you need and help others

Read Galatians 6:7-10. When we sow seeds from our sinful nature, what do we reap? What do we reap when we sow seeds from the Spirit?

destruction

Eternal Life

Seeds don't sprout and mature instantly. A farmer must work and toil for a good harvest. According to verses 9 and 10, how do we nurture the seeds of the Spirit to reap a harvest?

Keep doing good

How will you sow generously in the lives of those around you this week?

Dear Lord, Your grace is more wonderful than I can imagine. You supply my needs and continue to give me surpassing grace. Thank You. Amen.

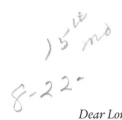

A POWERFUL RELATIONSHIP

Dear Lord, by Your grace I am saved and changed. May I use Your amazing gift to help others. Amen.

Water is not only necessary for life; it is also incredibly powerful. You need only look at a large waterfall to see that fast-flowing water is nearly unstoppable. Yet when that power is channeled right, it can be both beautiful and beneficial, as in the case of hydroelectic power plants. Niagara Falls is awe-inspiring to see, but it is also the largest producer of electricity for the State of New York. Energy from water is used all over the world to bring power to businesses and homes.

Grace is beautiful and necessary for life, but it is also astonishingly powerful. Grace changed Paul from a persecutor of Christians to a missionary. That's power. Let's look at the power grace brings into our lives so that we can be a light to those in darkness.

Read Ephesians 3:7-9. How was God's grace given to Paul (see verse 7)?

_____

_____

_____

In your own words, describe God's purpose in giving Paul His grace.

_____

_____

_____

_____

We, like Paul, are called to share Christ with those who need Him. What is keeping you from sharing your faith? What kind of power do you need to overcome those obstacles?

_____

_____

_____

In Ephesians 3:17-18, what kind of power did Paul pray we would receive?

The depth of God love

How might the power of knowing how immense Christ's love is enable you to share Him with others?

understanding Gods love for us

The power of Christ's grace helps us experience His love, for through that grace, we are able to discover the width, breadth and depth of God's love for us. When the power of God's grace works in us to reveal His love, we light up with knowledge of "the unsearchable riches of Christ" (Ephesians 7:8). Sharing that light will change the lives of those living in darkness.

> *Dear Lord, You bless me more each day with Your grace, power and love. Help me share You! Amen.*

Day 6 — REFLECTION AND APPLICATION

Dear Lord, You care enough to meet my needs daily. Thank You for all You do for me. Amen.

Marie was a stay-at-home mom for five children, and her husband was unemployed. His small pension wasn't much, but she was determined to make it stretch at home while he looked for steady work.

In addition to the seven mouths she had to feed every day, Marie's teen sons brought home friends whose parents weren't home in the evenings. She didn't have the heart to turn anyone away, especially lonely young people who just wanted to be with a family; so each morning when she made the dough for that evening's bread, she prayed that there would be enough for everyone at her table.

As the teens arrived in the evening, Marie added a potato to the oven or a helping of vegetables to the pot for each one, and then put the newcomer to work shaping bread loaves or setting the table, which let them know they were part of the family. This went on for months—and there was always enough. Everyone who came to Marie's table was filled. Every bill that was due got paid, sometimes from an unexpected source. And every night around the dinner table, Marie led the "family" in a prayer of thanks for God's provision.

We may not have a surplus, but we don't need to be anxious. God will provide for our needs as we seek to serve others through His grace.

Have you ever received an unexpected gift of money, food or other provision just when you needed it? What happened?

_____

_____

_____

_____

_____

When has God moved you to give food or money to someone who needed it? How did he or she react?

_____

_____

_____

_____

God provides for more than material needs. In 2 Timothy 2, Paul assured Timothy that God's grace would strengthen him by helping him develop patience, kindness and other qualities. Consider how God has also supplied non-material needs in your life. When have you been drained of energy and been refreshed by a Scripture or other encouragement?

_____

_____

_____

_____

When have you reaped more success than you expected?

_____

_____

_____

_____

How might remembering God's provision in the past help you remain confident during future hard times?

_____

_____

_____

_____

What is your greatest need right now? What, if anything, is keeping you from trusting God and letting go of worry?

_____

_____

_____

_____

As we learned from Ephesians 3:20 on Day 5, God is able to do exceedingly more abundantly beyond all that we ask. Expect answers and expect His help as you follow Him and work hard at whatever task He gives you.

Dear Lord, thank You for helping me be free of worry. Help me to trust Your grace to supply my needs. Amen.

REFLECTION AND APPLICATION

*Dear Lord, root me in Your love that I might grow to be more like You.
Nourish my mind and heart as I meditate on Your Word. Amen.*

As we read in Ephesians 3, God wants to give you the power of His grace to experience the fullness of His Son's love for you. Before that can happen, however, we must be "rooted and established in love" (verse 17). One of the best ways to sink our roots deep in God's love is to study the Scriptures, where God reveals Himself to us.

Good methods and tools will help you make the most of your daily study. A concordance is an invaluable tool that lists, in alphabetical order, the important words used most often in God's Word. You can look up the word "provide" or "strength" to see a list of all the Bible verses that contain that word.

A Bible dictionary can also be useful, by helping you understand what you read. Because Scripture was written many centuries ago in cultures very different from ours, it can sometimes be hard to understand. Likewise, maps can give you "big picture" insights into the places recorded in the Bible.

Before you get started with your daily study, pray that the Holy Spirit will open your mind and heart as you read. Then, as you read your chosen passage for the day, try to answer these questions: *Who wrote this? Who is it written to? What was happening at the time?* (A concordance, Bible dictionary and maps will come in handy as you discover the answers.) Then, once you understand the original context of the passage, think about how it applies to your own situation. *What can you learn? How can this knowledge help you grow?*

What is the best time(s) of day for you to read the Bible?

_____

_____

_____

_____

How long will you devote to reading and praying?

_____
_____
_____
_____
_____

How often will you write in your journal to record prayers, thoughts from God or verses you want to remember?

_____
_____
_____
_____
_____

What verses have brought you hope during a tough time?

_____
_____
_____
_____

What verses have given you comfort or strength?

_____
_____
_____
_____

What is your favorite Bible verse or passage? Why?

_____
_____
_____
_____

Make a plan to be more diligent in Bible study during the coming week. After seven days, spend some time thinking about how daily study is changing you. Can you see that you are more "rooted and established in love"?

Dear Lord, help me to be diligent in studying the Bible. Today, I pray that You would enlighten my mind and open my heart as I read Your Word. Thank You, Lord. Amen.

Notes

1. "The Importance of Water and Human Health," Water Education, FreeDrinking Water.com. http://www.freedrinkingwater.com/water-education/water-health.htm.
2. William Schafer and Shirley T. Munson, "Freezing Fruits and Vegetables," University of Minnesota, 2009. http://www.extension.umn.edu/distribution/nutrition/dj0555.html.

Group Prayer Requests

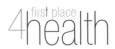

Today's Date: _____

Name	Request

Results

_____

_____

_____

_____

_____

Week Seven

---

connected
to grace

SCRIPTURE MEMORY VERSE

*I am the vine; you are the branches. If a man remains in me and I in him,
he will bear much fruit; apart from me you can do nothing.*

JOHN 15:5

Through the Internet, people have become connected in a new way. In seconds, messages cross thousands of miles to let people chat, shop, play or share information. Internet technology helps us feel as though we belong, connected to a network of relationships that spans the globe.

The Internet is a wonderful metaphor for the connectedness God wants us to experience with His people, the Church. Yet none of these connections with family and friends can compare to the connection we can have with Jesus, through His grace. His grace, unlike Internet devices, never breaks down. It doesn't require a computer or smart phone to access Him. Jesus is 100-percent reliable.

This week we will learn about our divine connections and find out how to stay close to Him.

CONNECTED TO THE SOURCE

Day
1

*Dear Lord, help me understand how to stay close to
You and how to bear fruit. Amen.*

Jesus used the image of a vine to illustrate our relationship with Him. One large root in the ground supports many branches and abundant clusters of grapes. The branches spread out and twist in many directions, all the while staying connected to the vine. He delivers the nutrients and energy we need to grow, supplying all of our needs so that we can bear fruit.

Read John 15:1-4. According to these verses, what is the relationship between you, the Father and Jesus?

we are all connected
We are a part of Him & He in us

What does the Father, the gardener, do?

prunes or disciplines.

21⁻19   12-5-10

11-2 Vine growers in Jesus' time used three main methods for pruning their vines. First, they pinched the tips of new shoots to slow their growth, making sure the new growth stayed close to the vine during its formative stages (up to three years). This is a vivid picture of how important it is for new Christians to stay close to the Vine, learning the Word and gathering their strength.

Second, vine growers "topped" larger branches to prevent them from becoming long and weak. A branch that used all its energy to grow away from the vine would not have enough energy to bear very much fruit. This picture shows us how important it is for maturing Christians to stay close to Christ, as well—that is how we will bear the fruit we are created to produce. We can also expect God's pruning to sometimes be painful. It may come in the form of sickness, relational breakdown or financial troubles; whatever shape it takes, we can be confident that these trials are God's way of preparing us to bear fruit.

Third, vine growers cut away dying branches and under-sized grape clusters. This allowed the nutrients sent out by the vine to strengthen the most productive branches. This picture is a warning to us: If we do not stay close to the Vine and produce all the fruit He desires for us, He will focus His power and strength on believers who will.[1]

Read John 15:5-8. Why is it important that a branch remain connected to the vine?

Apart from the vines you can do nothing.

According to verse 7, what two things must happen for us to receive what we need?

Remain in me & ask

According to verse 8, what does Jesus expect of you?

bear much fruit and show yourselves to be disciples

Turn to John 15:9-17. How can we remain in Jesus' love (see verses 10, 12 and 14)?

Love each other as I have loved you this is Jesus command

Dear Lord, thank You for being the vine that supplies all I need to grow. Amen.

MACEDONIAN EXAMPLE

Dear Lord, help me to grow in grace and produce fruit of generosity to help others. Amen.

Yesterday, we learned about being connected to Christ, the Vine, and bearing fruit. The apostle Paul, whose life's work was to help Christians learn how to do these things, pointed to the example of a group of Christians in Macedonia.

Read 2 Corinthians 8:1-5. What did God give the Macedonian church?

God gave them grace of giving

_____

_____

What fruits grew from the trials (pruning) they had experienced?

_____

_____

_____

After pointing to the Macedonians as models, Paul then turned his focus on the Corinthians. Titus had come from Corinth to give Paul a report of the church there. Turn to 2 Corinthians 8:6-7. What fruit was evidenced in the Corinthian Christians? What did Paul hope would increase in them?

_____

_____

_____

Read 2 Corinthians 8:8-15. How did Paul use Christ as an illustration of the grace of giving (see verses 8-9)?

_____

_____

_____

Although Paul praised the Corinthians for their desire to give, what did he challenge them to do (see verses 10-15)?

_____

_____

_____

_____

In verse 15, Paul refers to the manna that God sent daily to the Israelites when they wandered in the desert (see Exodus 16). What promise is implied in this verse for people who give generously?

_____

_____

_____

_____

_____

In a great network, everyone benefits. All benefit from the nourishment that Christ, the true Vine, provides. And all can be fruitful with an abundance that can be shared.

Dear Lord, help me to act on my desire to give generously. Help me trust that You will supply all I need no matter how much I give. Amen.

UNITY WITH GRACE

Day 3

Dear Lord, You are the Vine and I am united to You as a branch. Help me continue to grow and be united with other believers through You. Amen.

All the branches (believers) are connected to each other through the Vine (Christ). We share the blessings given by God's grace. In the Early Church, believers expressed this unity of heart and mind by sharing their possessions and providing for each others' needs. Let's look at how God's grace unified them.

Read Acts 4:32-37. How was unity expressed among the believers (see verse 32)?

_____

_____

_____

_____

How do you think the believers' generosity to one another was connected to their focus on Jesus' resurrection?

_____

_____

_____

_____

What did people do to prevent anyone from being needy (see verse 34)?

_____

_____

_____

_____

The Early Church began at Pentecost, when the Holy Spirit came just as Jesus had promised. Let's next look at the fellowship believers shared. According to Acts 2:41-47, how many became believers on the Day of Pentecost?

_____

_____

_____

_____

What resulted from the grace in their lives (see verse 47)?

_____

_____

_____

Describe the "heart condition" of those earliest believers. How did their actions reflect their hearts?

_____

_____

_____

How do you think being filled with awe and having a glad, sincere heart will have an impact on your actions? What can you do to cultivate this "heart condition" and unity with other believers?

_____

_____

_____

Dear Lord, I am amazed as I grow in knowledge of You. May Your grace overflow in my life in unity with other believers. Amen.

GRACE UPON GRACE   Day 4

Lord, You have blessed me with Your grace and salvation. You offer more blessings that are so wonderful. Amen.

We can expect unfathomable blessings when we stay connected to Christ, the Vine. Read John 1:16-18. The Law that God gave His people through Moses was a gift, but it could not compare to the blessings He gave through Jesus. What are those blessings?

_____

_____

_____

According to verse 18, what does Jesus' relationship to the Father allow us to do?

_____

_____

_____

What does it mean to you that you can personally know the Creator of the universe? What does that grace mean for your life and your situation?

_____

_____

_____

_____

Turn to Ephesians 1:2-9. Notice that in addition to material blessings, God also graces us with spiritual blessings through His Son. In your own words, summarize the spiritual benefits listed in verses 4 to 9.

_____

_____

_____

_____

_____

In Matthew 5:1-12, Jesus also promised that earthly problems would lead to blessings in eternity. In the following table, indicate what blessing He promised for each temporary problem.

Temporary problem	Promised blessing
The poor in spirit (those who trust God instead of themselves)	
Those who mourn (or grieve)	
The meek (those who are humble)	
Those who hunger and thirst for righteousness (or who seek justice)	
The merciful	

Temporary problem	Promised blessing
The pure in heart	
The peacemakers	
Those who arc persecuted because of righteousness	

Even the troubles and trials we experience here on earth will lead to unimaginable blessings from above!

Dear Lord, thank You for each blessing You give to me.
Help me to appreciate all that You do. Amen.

CONNECTING IN PRAYER

Day 5

Dear Lord, I want to be close to You and hear Your voice. Amen.

Prayer is a powerful connection to Jesus. Today, we will look at how Jesus is approachable and wants us to pray. We'll use the word P-R-A-Y-E-R as an acrostic to learn about various aspects of communicating with Him.

The **P** in P-R-A-Y-E-R is for *praise*. Read Revelation 5:11-12. Why is God worthy of praise?

_____

_____

_____

_____

When we praise, we are also reminded that God's power is greater than any problem we may face. In Mark 9:20-24, how did Jesus respond to a father's request for his son (see verse 23)? How can praising God remind you of this truth?

_____

_____

_____

_____

Praising God for His greatness and holiness also reminds us that we sin and need His forgiveness. The **R** in P-R-A-Y-E-R is for *repent*. According to 1 John 1:9 and Acts 3:19, what happens when we repent and admit our sins?

_____

_____

_____

_____

Praise and repentance put us in a right relationship with God. Next, we bring our needs before Him. The **A** in P-R-A-Y-E-R stands for *ask*. Read Jesus' words Matthew 21:21-22. What will happen if we believe? What does this mean for us?

_____

_____

_____

_____

According to Matthew 7:9-11, how do we know that God wants to answer our requests?

_____

_____

_____

_____

God wants to provide for our needs. However, He's not a genie who responds to our commands, especially when we demand things that aren't really needed. We are to yield to His will. The **Y** in P-R-A-Y-E-R stands for *yield*. Read 1 John 5:14-15. How should we ask?

_____

_____

_____

If we yield to God's will, we should expect to receive answers. The **E** in P-R-A-Y-E-R stands for *expect answers*. According to Matthew 7:7, what happens when we ask? What happens when we seek? What happens when we knock on heaven's door?

_____

_____

_____

God will respond, so we should always be listening for His reply. We also need to ready ourselves to respond when He directs us. The **R** in P-R-A-Y-E-R stands for *respond*. Read James 1:22. How should we respond when we read God's Word?

_____

_____

_____

_____

Let prayer become a habit that builds your relationship with God and keeps you connected to Jesus.

Dear Lord, thank You for always listening to my prayers.
Let prayer change me. Amen.

REFLECTION AND APPLICATION

Dear Lord, thank You for being my Source of indescribable grace. I am amazed by the wonders of Your works. Amen.

God answers prayer—sometimes in the most surprising ways. Even though He already knows our needs, He desires for us to pray regularly and diligently. Meeting with God every day in prayer builds our relationship with Him and prepares us to be used by Him when He answers our prayer. Today, we will review the P-R-A-Y-E-R acrostic we looked at yesterday and begin to put it into practice.

Praise God
Repent of sins
Ask for God's help
Yield to God's will
Expect answers
Respond to God's direction

P*raise.* Write a prayer of praise to God below in your own words or use a psalm of praise (such as Psalm 145) as a guide.

_____

_____

_____

_____

_____

R*epent.* List anything you have done this week that might have hurt others. Reflect on your list and ask God to show you where you need His forgiveness.

_____

_____

_____

_____

Ask. List some of your own needs and those of your loved ones.

_____

_____

_____

_____

_____

Yield. Are you willing to yield to God's will no matter the outcome? Write a note to Him expressing your desire to follow His will and not your own desires.

_____

_____

_____

_____

Expect answers. Paul's words in Philippians 4:6 provide a reminder for us to be joyful and give thanks while asking for God's help. We should be so prepared for God to answer that we can thank Him even before receiving the answer. Write a note of thanks for how He will answer your prayers and provide for your needs.

_____

_____

_____

_____

Respond. As we draw close to God in prayer, we can expect Him to guide us to meet others' needs, His commands or grow in some way. What is God directing you to do? How will you respond to Him?

_____

_____

_____

_____

_____

God is a God of grace who answers prayers. Trust your needs to Him and watch what He does.

Dear Lord, thank You for listening when I pray. I am ready for Your answer according to Your will. Amen.

Day 7 — REFLECTION AND APPLICATION

Lord Jesus, You are the Vine and I am a small branch. Help me as I am pruned to be more fruitful. Amen.

We have looked this week at what happens when we are connected to Christ, the Vine. We get to know the Father, we receive unimaginable blessings and we build relationships with others. One of the main goals, however, of a close connection to Christ is to bear fruit for Him! In Galatians 5:22-23, Paul lists this fruit of the Spirit: "The fruit of the Spirit is love, joy, peace, patience, kindness, goodness, faithfulness, gentleness and self-control."

In Matthew 7:20, Jesus says, "By their fruit you will recognize them." Are you recognizable as a child of God by the fruit your bear in your life? What fruit are you producing? What fruit needs more cultivation?

_____

_____

_____

_____

Being pruned is not fun. It hurts, but it helps us be more fruitful. God trims away our sins and stops us from growing in the wrong direction. What has God done to prune old habits and make you more fruitful?

_____

_____

_____

Think of a difficulty you are facing now. How might that be God's way of pruning you? How is it changing you?

_____

_____

_____

_____

_____

Is it hard for you to see your pain or discomfort as loving discipline from God? How might viewing your trials in this way help you to endure (see Hebrews 12:7-11)?

_____

_____

_____

_____

_____

We can have hope in hardship because we know it means God is pruning us, nurturing new growth in us. We can also rejoice that we are part of such a great network of people, all connected to the Vine!

> *Dear Father, thank You for caring enough to make me stronger.*
> *Help me endure the pruning and learn from it. Amen.*

Note

1. J.D. Douglas, et. al, eds., *The New Bible Dictionary* (Downers Grove, IL: InterVarsity Press, 1982), pp. 1236-1237.

Group Prayer Requests

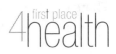

Today's Date: _____

Name	Request

Results

_____

_____

_____

_____

_____

_____

strengthened by grace

SCRIPTURE MEMORY VERSE

The name of the Lord is a strong tower; the righteous run to it and are safe.

PROVERBS 18:10

In ancient times, towers were an important part of a city's military defenses. People surrounded their cities with strong walls to keep enemies out and incorporated towers, often at the corners, to provide protection for the lookouts. Towers also served as strategic places from which to shoot arrows at an attacker and a refuge of last resort if the walls failed.

In the Bible, the tower metaphor is sometimes used to emphasize God's character; He watches over and protects His people, and provides for their needs. In times of great trouble, God's people run to Him for safety. The word "safe" in this week's memory verse is the Hebrew word *sâgab*, which means "lofty." The implication is that God will lift up His people, out of evil's reach, whenever they run to Him.

This week we'll look at God as the one who protects us and strengthens us by His grace. We'll also study how we can "run to Him" in prayer.

OLD TESTAMENT TOWERS
Day 1

Father God, You are my fortress and tower at all times.
Protect me and guard me from harm. Amen.

One of the most famous towers from biblical history is the Tower of Babel (see Genesis 11:1-9). When the ancient people got together to build it, their goal was to become so powerful that they would not need God. The Tower of Babel, and other biblical examples of humankind's arrogance, stands in stark contrast to the picture of God as our unfailing tower. Let's compare the unreliability of manmade "towers," such as wealth, pride and reputation, with the faithfulness of God.

Read Proverbs 18:10-12. According to verse 11, what do the rich imagine their wealth provides?

_____

_____

_____

What does verse 12 imply will happen to the proud?

_____

_____

What happens to people who run to God as their tower instead of trusting in wealth or pride?

_____

_____

_____

Look up Genesis 35:21. Where did Jacob (called Israel) pitch his tent?

_____

_____

Now turn to Micah 4:8. What is this tower called?

_____

_____

Migdal is Hebrew for "tower," while *Eder* means "flock." These two verses are referring to the same place: the watchtower of the flock, or Migdal Eder. This tower stood somewhere near Bethlehem, on the road to Jerusalem. From its heights, watchmen kept a lookout over the special flocks used for Temple sacrifices. Its mention in Micah 4 is a prophecy about the coming Messiah, Jesus, who would be sacrificed to save us, once and for all. Long before His birth, God was keeping watch. As you think about God's plan to save His people—to save you—what are your thoughts about His faithfulness?

_____

_____

_____

God watches over us, and we can run to Him in times of trouble. He is always faithful to save us. He is also the source of our provision, supplying our every need from His limitless storehouse of blessing. What kind of tower do you need God to be today? Do you need protection? Salvation? Provision? Write a short prayer asking God to be your strong Tower.

_____

_____

_____

Heavenly Father, You are my Tower of protection, my storehouse of provisions and my place of refuge where I can come in prayer. Amen.

GRACE FOR THE RACE

Day 2

Dear Father, let me run to You in confidence, knowing that You are ready to protect me. Make my path straight. Amen.

Our ability to "run to the tower" is dependent on two things: (1) that we are physically fit enough to run, and (2) that we know where the tower is located. The implication is that we must get these two factors in order *before* danger comes, so that we do not spend precious time searching for the tower or stopping to catch our breath! The apostle Paul understood how important it is to know where we are headed, and he used the metaphor of running a race to illustrate the importance of training.

Read 1 Corinthians 9:24-27. Why do we run the race?

_____
_____
_____

What should we do to prepare ourselves to run?

_____
_____
_____

The author of Hebrews also understood the importance of knowing our goal. According to Hebrews 12:1-3, where should our eyes be fixed?

_____
_____
_____

According to verse 1, what two things should we do to run the race God has marked out for us?

_____
_____
_____

In First Place 4 Health, we strive for a better physical body. How does the work you do to be more balanced and fit help you understand the metaphor of a race?

_____
_____
_____

There are times when we feel tired and worn out, unable to keep running. But we can have hope to endure. Turn to Isaiah 40:28-31. What will happen as we hope in the Lord?

_____

_____

_____

_____

God is our source of strength who will help us press on when we feel tired. As we keep our eyes fixed on Him, He will renew our energy.

Dear Lord, help me keep my eyes on You so that I may finish the race that is before me. Amen.

MORE GRACE

Day 3

Dear Father, give me grace for today to run and not grow weary. Help me to run for the right prize. Amen.

As we realize that all we have is from God, our response should be humility. We cannot protect ourselves with wealth or pride; giving generously of our resources can remind us of our dependence on God's grace. Today, we will look at the pitfalls of self-reliance and how to have the right attitude toward money.

In Luke 12:15-21, Jesus told a story about a proud man who built his own storehouse only to discover that hoarding wealth was all in vain. What did the man in this story do when he was blessed with an abundant crop? How did he plan to live based on his wealth?

_____

_____

_____

_____

How did God respond to the man's plans?

_____

_____

_____

Jesus said, "This is how it will be with anyone who stores up things for himself but is not rich toward God" (verse 21). What does it mean to be "rich toward God"?

_____

_____

_____

We can learn more about being "rich toward God" from instructions the apostle Paul gave to his young friend Timothy. Read 1 Timothy 6:10-19. What should we flee from? What should we pursue (see verse 11)?

_____

_____

_____

It is not a sin to be wealthy; in fact, God stands ready to bless those who are generous with even more resources. But how should the rich live (see verses 17-19)?

_____

_____

_____

When we see people around us who have more than we do, it is tempting to think of ourselves as "poor." But in comparison to the many millions of people who live in extreme poverty, we are rich indeed! According to Matthew 6:31-34, what should our attitude be toward our needs?

_____

_____

_____

What can we trust that God will do when we seek Him first?

_____

_____

_____

Father, help me to seek You first each day and trust You to meet my needs.

OUR TOWER AND FORTRESS
God, strengthen me with grace for all You want me to do. Amen.

Day 4

God is our tower of strength, our mighty fortress. Up until some centuries ago, fortresses were a necessary part of a city's defenses. A fortress had thick, high walls and was usually built on a hill or outcropping that commanded a view of the city. The fortress was the first line of defense and the last refuge for people under siege. Let's look today at how God, our tower and fortress, strengthens His people.

Read Psalm 28:6-8. How does God respond to those who come to Him for mercy?

_____

_____

_____

What type of fortress is God?

_____

_____

_____

According to Colossians 1:10-12, why does God give us strength? Why do we need strength for endurance and patience?

_____

_____

_____

Turn to 2 Thessalonians 3:3. What will God strengthen and protect us from? In what area do you need protection from temptation in your life right now?

_____

_____

_____

According to Deuteronomy 31:6, how does God's presence strengthen you?

_____

_____

_____

Read Psalm 119:28-32. How does God's Word strengthen you?

_____

_____

_____

God's Word is a source of His grace. Reading and meditating on His Word help us in times of sorrow and help us discern deceit. He gives us His laws to guide us, not to make us slaves to rules, just as parents set rules to keep their children safe. That God is watching over us and His presence is with us should give us courage and hope. The hope strengthens our hearts and reminds us that we don't have to face problems alone.

Dear Father, thank You for being with me as my constant source of grace and strength. Amen.

Day 5 — REMAIN STRONG IN GRACE

Dear Lord, strengthen me with grace and remain with me as I face today. Amen.

When young children are afraid, their father picks them up and wraps his strong arms around them. His presence, protection and love calm their fears and let them know that they are safe. Likewise, our heavenly

Father lifts us into His arms when we feel afraid, protecting us from anything that might cause us harm. Let's look at two psalms that reveal how God protects us.

Read Psalm 61:4-8. Why do you think the psalmist asks God for His love and faithfulness, rather than His power and might, to protect him (see verse 7)?

_____

_____

_____

What should be our response to God's faithful protection (see verse 8)?

_____

_____

_____

Turn to Psalm 91:1-8. How is God's protection described (see verses 3-4)?

_____

_____

_____

When we are confident of God's protection, we can have courage. When we focus on God and His limitless ability, we can breathe deep and feel secure. Rewrite verses 5-7 in your own words.

_____

_____

_____

Read Psalm 91:9-13. These verses tell us how safe we are under God's care. What happens when we make the Most High our dwelling place?

_____

_____

_____

Because of God's great love for you, He wants to protect and save you. How has God protected you in the past? In what situation do you need God's protection and salvation in the future?

_____

_____

_____

When we recall God's past protection, it is easier to trust Him for present and future needs. Trust that God will be your strong Tower always. Imagine Him as a loving Father reaching out and lifting you up with strong arms.

Dear Father, I am so thankful for Your loving protection and strength. Amen.

Day 6 — REFLECTION AND APPLICATION

Dear Father, give me strength in mind, body and soul. Help me face the challenges of each day. Amen.

Darlene stopped at a red light on her way home from teen choir practice. Unfortunately, an approaching truck did not stop—it rammed into her at 40 miles an hour. Her wounded body healed after some time and therapy, but her mind was bound by post-traumatic stress. Before the accident, Darlene had been able to focus on her studies and remember facts easily, but now she struggled to master her classes, especially history.

Darlene's mom tried to tutor her, helping as much as she could, but nothing seemed to help. At their wits' end, they prayed together that Darlene's mind would be healed. After several days, Darlene's mom suggested that they take a walk while talking about history. At first it sounded to both of them like a strange idea, but they both felt that study-walking was what God was leading them to do. There was an 8-mile walking path behind their home that wound around tree-lined lakes, so Darlene and her mom set out.

As they walked and talked about history, Darlene began to grasp the ideas and facts that had been eluding her. Slowly, by walking a little farther each day, she regained her focus and memory. It made sense: Darlene was a kinesthetic learner who learned best when she was *doing*, not just talking! Study-walking not only improved her history grades, but it also finished the healing of her body. In addition, her mom lost some stubborn weight, too. Even after the school year ended, Darlene and her mom continued to walk, praying and talking as they went.

When we pray, God often impresses a solution on our minds that becomes the answer to our prayers. Rather than "magically" changing the situation, He shows us how we can work with Him to answer our prayers.

What struggles are most on your heart when you run to God in prayer?

_____

_____

_____

Have you prayed for God's grace to help you face the problem? If so, what has God shown you that *you* can do to work with Him in answering your prayer?

_____

_____

_____

What has worked for you in the First Place 4 Health program?

_____

_____

_____

What unexpected blessings have you received while following the program?

_____

_____

_____

Grace upon grace is something God wants to give us. Take time each morning to ask God for grace for the day. Each evening, reflect on how God gave you grace.

Dear Lord, thank You for Your grace each day and for helping me with my struggles. Allow me to see the unexpected blessings You also give me. Amen.

Day 7

REFLECTION AND APPLICATION

Dear Lord, give me strength each day for my mind, body, soul and emotions. Help me have the strength to say no to temptations and to say yes to Your plans for me. Amen.

Progress, not perfection, is the goal of First Place 4 Health and of the Christian life. Hopefully, you have been asking God for grace to work toward balance in each of the four areas of your life. Change takes time, and every little step or measure of progress is worth celebrating. For each area of your life, list your needs, improvements and how God's grace has helped you make progress.

Mental

_____
_____
_____
_____
_____

Emotional

_____
_____
_____
_____
_____

Spiritual

_____

_____

_____

_____

Physical

_____

_____

_____

_____

Which area needs the most work? Why?

_____

_____

_____

Paul had strict training for himself. That means scheduling time and sticking to it. What times have you set for the following?

Bible study: _____

Prayer: _____

Exercise: _____

Planning your menu: _____

Review how God's grace has given you strength so far in this session, and write a short prayer thanking Him for His faithfulness.

_____

_____

_____

Dear Lord, may Your grace continue to strengthen my body, mind, heart and soul. Give me grace to continue with this plan. Amen.

Group Prayer Requests

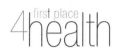

Today's Date: _____

Name	Request

Results

_____

_____

_____

_____

_____

_____

living in
grace

SCRIPTURE MEMORY VERSE

*So then, just as you received Christ Jesus as Lord, continue to
live in him, rooted and built up in him, strengthened in the faith
as you were taught, and overflowing with thankfulness.*

COLOSSIANS 2:6-7

A study conducted by researchers at the University of California, Davis, and the University of Miami identified several positive benefits of keeping a "gratitude journal."[1] Thankful people reported feeling happier, more alert and more optimistic, and were more likely to help others. They also felt more loved.

When we give thanks, we meditate on something positive that has happened to us, rather than focusing on something negative. It makes sense that this would have an impact on our attitude! Expressing thanks acknowledges God's blessings and the role others have played in our lives, which help us to respond with kind actions.

God's grace is reason enough to give thanks, but it turns out that giving thanks brings further blessings! Let's look at the examples of biblical men and women who expressed their thanks and were blessed.

GRACE THAT INSPIRES THANKSGIVING   Day 1

Dear Lord, Your grace fills my heart, and I praise You for Your blessings. Amen.

Jesus spoke about the connection between forgiveness and gratitude when a woman forgiven of great sins washed His feet with her tears and dried them with her hair. Her heart overflowed with so much gratitude that she couldn't keep from continually kissing His feet. A Pharisee watching the woman reacted with contempt, but Jesus pointed to the woman as an example of love and forgiveness. Today, we will look at this unnamed woman and the relationship between grace and gratitude.

Read Luke 7:36-50. How is the woman's life described (see verse 37)?

_____

_____

_____

_____

_____

What did the woman do for Jesus? How did the Pharisee react?

_____

_____

_____

_____

Summarize, in your own words, the story that Jesus told Simon, the Pharisee.

_____

_____

_____

_____

_____

How did Jesus contrast the kind actions of the woman with Simon's?

_____

_____

_____

_____

_____

According to Jesus, what made the difference in their actions (see verse 47)?

_____

_____

_____

_____

Everyone has sinned, and all sin is unholy to God. Jesus died for every person and loves us all the same. But some people try to justify their actions and consider their sins less severe than someone else's. They do this to feel better about themselves, but this attitude keeps their heart from the gratefulness that comes when they truly acknowledge the cost of forgiveness. In verse 50, we read that Jesus gave the woman a blessing of peace. Do you think Simon received the same blessing? Why or why not?

_____

_____

_____

_____

How are thankfulness and peace connected? Why might someone who is grateful experience peace?

_____

_____

_____

Are you in need of peace? Try giving thanks, especially for all you have been forgiven. Spend a few minutes thinking about the blessings for which you are thankful, including God's forgiveness. See if you experience peace as you remind yourself of God's grace.

Dear Lord, thank You for dying for me and blessing me with grace.
Help me focus on You and not on my circumstances. Amen.

HANNAH'S GRATITUDE

Dear Father, help me develop an attitude of gratitude. You have made the earth and filled it with wonders and blessed me with Your love. Thank You. Amen.

The heart of one woman in the Old Testament, Hannah, changed from sorrow to contentment as she poured out her pain in prayer. Read 1 Samuel 1:2-18. What caused Hannah to feel sad? How did her husband respond (see verses 4-8)?

_____

_____

_____

It is never easy to live with an unanswered prayer. How did Hannah react to her problem (see verses 10-11)?

_____

_____

_____

What did Eli, the priest, think Hannah had been doing? How did she respond (see verses 13-16)?

_____

_____

_____

_____

According to verse 18, how did Hannah's attitude, appetite and face change as she left the Temple? Why do you think she was changed?

_____

_____

_____

Continue reading the story in 1 Samuel 1:19-28. How did God respond to Hannah's prayer (see verse 19)?

_____

_____

_____

What did Hannah do after having her son?

_____

_____

_____

In 1 Samuel 2:1-10, Hannah sang a song of praise and thanks. What are some reasons she found to thank God?

_____

_____

_____

Hannah didn't ask for another child, even though she had given up her only son. She no longer focused on herself, but on God. Her heart overflowed with praise. If you have unanswered prayers, don't give up. Ask God to change your attitude, and pray for contentment in the midst of your need.

Lord, help me find contentment instead of worry, anger or sorrow.
Fill my heart with grace that I might overflow with gratitude. Amen.

GRATEFUL HEARTS AND KIND ACTIONS Day 3

Dear Lord, thank You for all the blessings You give. Help me to remember my blessings with gratitude. Amen.

Gratitude can cause us to act with kindness. King David felt such gratitude for his beloved friend Jonathan that he looked for a way to continue expressing his thanks long after Jonathan had died. Read 2 Samuel 9:1-8. Why did David want to find someone from Jonathan's family? Who did he find?

_____

_____

_____

_____

What problem did Jonathan's son have (see verse 3)?

_____

_____

_____

Jonathan had been in line for the throne of Israel, and his surviving son was his heir. Because of this, Mephibosheth could have been a rival to David. Despite this, what did David do for Jonathan's son?

_____

_____

_____

_____

According to 2 Thessalonians 2:13-17, how can grace encourage us to do good deeds (actions of kindness)?

_____

_____

_____

What has God given us (see verse 16)? How does remembering what God has done help us feel grateful?

_____

_____

_____

How can gratitude strengthen your heart?

_____

_____

_____

_____

_____

Studies have shown that there is a connection between grateful hearts and kind actions. A heart that is filled with love and thankfulness spills over in kind words and deeds. Make time daily to express gratitude toward God and others.

Dear Lord, strengthen my heart and show me good deeds I can do. Help my lips praise You and overflow with kindness toward others. Amen.

COMMITTED TO GOD AND HIS GRACE   Day 4

Dear Lord, I want to be loving and giving. Strengthen me to look to the needs of others and to trust Your grace to provide for my needs. Amen.

Paul committed his life to reaching people with the gospel, helping the weak, and spreading God's grace that had so changed his life. He spent three years in Ephesus discipling the new church there. When the time came for him to depart, he gave his final farewell with some words of wisdom that encouraged giving—a giving that flowed from a thankful heart.

Read Acts 20:32-36 and write out the first 13 words of verse 32. What did Paul say grace could do?

_____

_____

_____

_____

_____

Paul had lived in Ephesus for three years, where his example showed the people his own commitment to Christ. This included showing his gratitude and his attitude toward giving. What had Paul shown them about living and money through his example?

_____

_____

_____

_____

What message did Paul give them from Jesus?

_____

_____

_____

_____

How does giving show our commitment to Christ?

_____

_____

_____

After Paul left another group of Christians, the Thessalonians, he sent them a letter with a message about love that flowed from thankfulness. Read 1 Thessalonians 3:9,11-13. What did Paul say about his thankfulness regarding the Thessalonians?

_____

_____

_____

_____

What is Paul's prayer to God for their hearts?

_____

_____

_____

Paul's unlimited thankfulness increased the love he felt for the Thessalonians. Thankfulness overflows into loving actions and through the actions people see our faith. Read John 13:34-35. What did Christ ask us to do?

_____

_____

_____

_____

Our connection to Christ will be evident in our love that flows from hearts thankful for the grace God has given us. Express gratitude to God and others today.

> _Dear Lord, I commit myself to You. I trust You with my life and_
> _ask You to direct me. Amen._

HEART OF GRATITUDE

Day 5

Dear Lord, when my courage fails and my heart fills with sorrow, I will
hope in You. Gracious Father, hear my cries and answer me. Amen.

When our heart is full of sorrow, we can become fearful or depressed. David, a man after God's own heart, struggled with fear and depression. In Psalm 31, he provides several reminders of God's greatness and other reasons to be thankful for God. This psalm can help us realize that God understands our hearts and will assist us as we persevere and hope in Him. Let's look at this psalm today and examine how David turned to God's grace for strength.

Begin today's study by reading Psalm 31. In verses 1-3, for what did David ask?

_____

_____

_____

How did David describe his condition (see verses 10-13)?

_____

_____

_____

_____

David's problems caused him inner anguish, physical illness, unhealthy weight loss and the slander and disrespect of those around him. Things couldn't get much worse! But what did David say that he hoped for (see verses 6-18,14-19)?

_____

_____

_____

_____

_____

Even in the midst of his dark days, David remembered God's goodness. And once he recalled God's goodness, he praised God and remembered to trust Him for the future. His gratefulness changed his attitude about his circumstances. In verses 23-24, what challenge did David offer to other saints who are hurting?

_____

_____

_____

_____

Now turn to Psalm 27:7,13-14. What themes do these verses echo from Psalm 31?

_____

_____

_____

_____

What is the hope found in Psalm 27:13? What does this mean to you in your particular circumstances?

_____

_____

_____

_____

_____

Read Psalm 28:6-9. How is the Lord described in these verses?

_____

_____

_____

_____

What happens when we trust in Him (see verse 7)?

_____

_____

_____

_____

Just when things can't get any worse—*that* is the time to give thanks! In Psalm 28:7, David wrote that his heart "leaps for joy" and that he would "give thanks to [the Lord] in song." Spend a few minutes writing your own psalm of thanks. Then, when times get tough, revisit your words. Lift your thanks to God and put your hope in Him!

_____

_____

_____

_____

_____

Heavenly Father, my hope is in You. Strengthen my heart and help me wait patiently. I thank You for all You have done. Amen.

REFLECTION AND APPLICATION

Dear Lord, thank You for all the grace You give me each day. Help me to have a heart that is filled with gratefulness. Amen.

On Day 2, we studied the life of Hannah, whose life was changed when she began to thank God. Let's see if we can apply Hannah's prayer method to our own circumstances.

Read 1 Samuel 2:1-10. List some of the reasons why Hannah thanked God.

_____

_____

_____

_____

Now list some of the reasons you are thankful.

_____

_____

_____

_____

Next, list some of God's attributes for which you are thankful.

_____

_____

_____

_____

How have you celebrated God's answers to prayer? What can you do to share how God has blessed you?

_____

_____

_____

_____

Kind actions flow from a grateful heart. How has someone acted kindly toward you in a way that showed he or she had a grateful heart? What actions have you done that flowed from being thankful?

_____

_____

_____

_____

The more you spend time expressing gratitude, the more your heart will respond with gratefulness for small and large blessings. Thinking of reasons to be grateful develops an awareness of all God's gifts.

> *Dear Lord, I rejoice as I review all Your answers to prayer. Help me to remember Your grace and respond with thanksgiving. Amen.*

REFLECTION AND APPLICATION

Day 7

> *Dear Lord, I am grateful for Your love, for friends, for family, for work, for Your creation and mostly for my salvation. Amen.*

Today, we are going to reflect on one line from 1 Corinthians 1:4-5: "I always thank God for you because of his grace given you in Christ Jesus. For in him you have been enriched in every way—in all your speaking and in all your knowledge." Being happy that God has blessed someone else can be difficult. It is tempting to be envious of another person's blessings. Paul attributes *all* blessings to God, which keeps the focus in the right place.

Who have you noticed who is rich in good speech, in words that sprinkle joy into others' lives, or in giving wisdom to those who need it?

_____

_____

_____

Who do you know to be rich in knowledge, in intelligence that gives insight to others, or in practical ways that help people get things done?

_____

_____

_____

_____

When was the last time you sent someone a thank-you note? What was it for? When was the last time you received a thank-you note? What was it for?

_____

_____

_____

_____

Paul usually followed his greeting with a blessing of grace to the recipient. How wonderful to bless the person you are writing to and impart God's grace to them! Paul often then followed this blessing with thanks, expressing his appreciation for the person or people to whom he was writing for their love and good work. For what will you thank someone? How can you bless that person with your words?

_____

_____

_____

_____

The heart of Paul's letters addressed issues or information that he wanted to share, describing what was happening in Paul's life and offering words of wisdom from his heart. What is on your heart to share with this person?

_____

_____

_____

Paul closed his letters with encouragement and inspiring thoughts. He usually ended with another blessing of peace and grace. How would you like to close your letter?

_____

_____

_____

_____

_____

Whether you send an email, an online instant message or a handwritten note by "snail mail," express your gratitude for someone today!

Dear Father, thank You for Your great love letter, the Bible. Help me have the words to write to my friend to pass on the blessings of Your grace. Amen.

Note

1. Robert A. Emmons and Michael E. McCullough, "Highlights from the Research Project on Gratitude and Thankfulness." http://psychology.ucdavis.edu/labs/emmons/ (accessed May 2010).

Group Prayer Requests

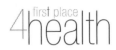

Today's Date: _____

Name	Request

Results

_____
_____
_____
_____
_____

responding in grace

SCRIPTURE MEMORY VERSE
*And whatever you do, whether in word or deed, do it all in the name
of the Lord Jesus, giving thanks to God the Father through Him.*
COLOSSIANS 3:17

Being mindful, or intentional, means to be focused and attentive or aware. This week's memory verse advises that all our actions should be done in the name of Jesus and with gratitude. To accomplish this, we must be mindful of our actions and intentional about giving Him thanks. When we practice this level of intentionality, we focus on God's power instead of our problems.

There are numerous examples from the Bible of people who lived mindfully and responded gratefully. These models show us how to put our trust in God and to reach out in grace to help His people.

ESTHER, A WOMAN OF GRACE

Day
1

*Dear Lord, help me to focus on You and choose to do Your will.
Thank You for Your grace in every situation. Amen.*

We don't often associate concern for others with beauty contestants, yet Esther, who became a queen when she won a beauty contest, put her own safety at risk to save her people. She put her trust in God and did what she knew was right, even when it could have meant her death. Let's discover more about Esther's example.

Read Esther 2. What had happened to Esther (see verse 7)? What information was she keeping secret (see verses 10,20)?

_____

_____

_____

_____

_____

The Jews who lived in Persia were foreigners and were not well respected in that country. It's likely that Mordecai wanted to help keep Esther safe by instructing her not to divulge her ethnicity and religion. Why was this good advice (see verse 15)?

_____

_____

_____

_____

There was one Persian noble who hated the Jews and devised a plot to annihilate them. Haman tricked the king, Xerxes, into issuing a decree that all the Jews should be destroyed. Read Esther 4:8-14. When Mordecai asked Esther to help, what was her first reaction?

_____

_____

_____

_____

What did Mordecai say to convince Esther to help (see verses 13-14)?

_____

_____

_____

_____

Esther knew that she was taking her life in her hands by going to the king without his permission, yet she knew that she must act. However, Esther took her time bringing her petition before the king—she asked him to a banquet, she "wined and dined" him, and then she asked him to return for another meal the following day. What does this reveal about intentionality?

_____

_____

_____

_____

Read Esther 8:3-6. How did Esther plead with the king on her people's behalf?

_____

_____

_____

_____

_____

While you are probably not facing a situation as dire as the Jews in Susa, there are probably people around you who need your help. Is it possible that God has placed you exactly where you are "for such a time as this"? What has He uniquely gifted you to do?

_____

_____

_____

As you become more willing to trust your future to God, He will use you in miraculous ways to impact others' lives.

Gracious Father, give me grace, courage and a humble spirit so that I might help others. Amen.

A CHURCH FULL OF GRACE

*Dear Lord, help me step out in faith, with Your grace. Let my actions
show Your grace at work. Amen.*

Yesterday we looked at the life of Esther, who put her trust in God's grace
and acted, at risk to her own life, in His name to save others. Today, let's
look at what happened when a group of Christians acted together to build
the Church. Read Acts 13:1-4. What let the church at Antioch know that
God wanted Barnabas and Saul (Paul) to set out on a missionary journey?

What did the people do before letting the men depart?

Their journey took Paul and Barnabas to several places. According to
Acts 14:1-3, how did God confirm His grace in Paul and Barnabas?

Acts 14: 26 in *THE MESSAGE* version reads, "Finally, they made it to At-
talia and caught a ship back to Antioch, where it had all started—
launched by God's grace and now safely home by God's grace. A good
piece of work." Imagine that you are a church member in Antioch. How
would you receive the news of Paul and Barnabas's journey?

While only Paul and Barnabas set out on the missionary journey, they went with the blessing and prayers of the entire church at Antioch. What difference do you think their support made for Paul and Barnabas's journey?

_____

_____

_____

_____

When have you participated in missionary work in person or by financial support and prayer? What impact did your support have on the work? How did the experience impact you?

_____

_____

_____

_____

God calls us to act in Christ's name. We can do that by acting as a team and being mindful of one another's purpose and needs.

Dear Lord, I'm so thankful that we are all one family, working together for Your purpose. Show me where I fit in and how I can help. Amen.

STEPHEN, A MAN FULL OF GRACE

Day 3

Dear Lord, help me follow You no matter the cost. I trust that Your grace will be enough for all I am called to do. Amen.

A Christian named Stephen became the first person to die for his faith in Christ. Right until the minute of his death, Stephen kept his mind on Christ and the needs of other people. Let's follow Stephen's example to discover how to act in grace.

Read Acts 6:1-15. What was Stephen's first task in the Early Church? Why was it important?

_____

_____

_____

_____

_____

Stephen served those in need, but God gave him additional gifts. What did God equip Stephen to do (see verse 8)?

_____

_____

_____

_____

_____

What happened to Stephen as a result of the work he was doing (see verses 9-15)?

_____

_____

_____

_____

_____

Acts 7 records a long speech Stephen gave before the council, testifying to the truth of Abraham, Moses, Joshua and David. Stephen ended by accusing the leaders of murdering Jesus, the Messiah. Read Acts 7:54-60. How did those in the court respond to Stephen's message?

_____

_____

_____

_____

As they stoned and killed Stephen, what did he say (see verse 56)?

_____

_____

_____

_____

Full of God's grace and power, Stephen set an example of doing tasks, both great and small, for the glory of God. Whether he was distributing food to needy widows or speaking prophetically before a crowd of hostile leaders, Stephen did his work in Jesus' name. What "small" tasks are before you today? How can you do them in Jesus' name?

_____

_____

_____

_____

Do you sense God's call to accomplish something "great"? How are you cultivating humility so that you will be prepared to do it in His name?

_____

_____

_____

_____

God may call you to do anything. As Stephen passed out food to widows, he may never have imagined that he would one day testify before the high priest or that his testimony would be recorded for all people and time. Instead, he focused on the "small" task before him, trusting the grace of God to provide future opportunities.

Dear Lord, thank You for every opportunity You give.
Help me follow You and do all things in Your name. Amen.

PURPOSE WITH GRACE

Dear Lord, You have a purpose for my life. Give me the grace to carry it out cheerfully. Help me to be strong and to follow You and Your plans. Amen.

In Stephen, we saw a man full of grace equipped with gifts of performing wonders and miracles. Throughout the New Testament, we find men and women equipped with various gifts, which God intended them to use in concert with other believers' gifts. As each Christian adds his or her gift to the Body of Christ, the Church is able to accomplish God's purpose: redeeming the world through His Son. Let's look at the spiritual gifts God gives and how we can use them in His grace as part of a team.

Read 1 Peter 4:7-16. Before Peter gave instructions to those with specific spiritual gifts, what three things did he command everyone to do (see verses 7-8)?

_____

_____

_____

The first spiritual gift Peter addressed is hospitality (see verse 9). How can hospitality help the Church accomplish God's purpose?

_____

_____

_____

_____

The next spiritual gift that Peter addressed is speaking (see verse 11), which could also be preaching or prophesying. How does this spiritual gift help accomplish God's purpose?

_____

_____

_____

_____

Finally, Peter addressed those with the spiritual gift of serving (see verse 11). While every Christian is called to serve, those with the gift of service have a special calling. How does this gift help accomplish God's purpose?

_____

_____

_____

_____

_____

As we contribute our spiritual gifts to the Church's mission, we should not be surprised when we face hardship. According to verses 12-16, how should we react when we suffer for Christ's sake?

_____

_____

_____

_____

_____

What should we commit to do in spite of suffering (see verse 19)?

_____

_____

_____

_____

_____

We can rejoice in our sufferings because of God's grace, continue in His purpose using our spiritual gifts and comfort one another with His love. Isn't that a beautiful picture of Christ's Body?

> _Dear Lord, today I pray that you would show me how to_
> _use my gifts and give me the courage to use them for Your glory._
> _Help me to face suffering with rejoicing. Amen._

BLESSED BY OUR GRACIOUS GOD

*Dear Father, You are for me so I know no one can oppose me. Bless me as I
follow Your will. Amen.*

Newton's Third Law of Motion states that every action causes an equal
and opposite reaction. While God is not subject to the physical laws that
govern our world, a similar principle is at work when we act in His grace:
As we act for God in word and deed, God responds. God longs to extend
grace to us and does so in response to our actions and faith. And when
we respond with praise and thanks, He blesses us all the more.

Read Isaiah 30:18-21. What does God long to do?

_____

_____

_____

If you listen, what will you hear (see verse 21)?

_____

_____

_____

Turn to Romans 8:28-39. If you are following God and serving His purpose, what can you expect in any circumstance (see verse 28)?

_____

_____

_____

What can separate you from God's love (see verse 35)? How do you respond to this knowledge?

_____

_____

_____

_____

Now read Numbers 6:22-27. This blessing is often used as a benediction in church services, even today. What does it mean to you that God's face is turned toward you, shining on you like the sun shines on the earth?

_____

_____

_____

According to Psalm 67:2, when God's face shines on us, what happens?

_____

_____

_____

The opening verses of this psalm request God's gracious blessings. The ending verses share how God blesses the people who praise Him. What is the purpose of the blessings?

_____

_____

_____

_____

God's grace and His blessings form a continuing circle of love, as we respond to Him in praise.

> *Dear Father, be gracious to me. Hear my cries when I am distressed and answer me. Send me mentors to help me along the way. Amen.*

REFLECTION AND APPLICATION

Dear Lord, guide me in responding to Your grace that I might help others in need. Amen.

Day 6

George Müller was put in prison at the age of 16 for defrauding an innkeeper. His life of sinful pleasure continued even after he was released, until his conversion at the age of 22. He turned around his life of crime when he attended a prayer meeting and saw a man on his knees in prayer. He heard the gospel for the first time and prayed for salvation, and became a Christian evangelist.

In his twenties, George moved from Germany to England, where he began his pastoral work. One of his main projects was to build and run orphanages for homeless children. When he began, he had only two shillings in his pocket, yet he trusted that God would provide for all his needs as long as he was seeking to spread His grace.

God did just that for more than 60 years. One remarkable time, the children gathered at the table for breakfast. Their bowls were empty and there was no food in the house. George bowed his head and thanked God for the food He would provide. Within minutes, a baker arrived with enough fresh bread for all the children, explaining that God had put it on his heart as he woke to bake it for them. Minutes later, a milk truck broke down in the street in front of the house. The milkman unloaded his truck to repair it and brought the milk inside for the children.

Similar needs were met without George ever having to mention them to anyone—he just prayed, and waited on God's provision. Years later, George reflected on his life and the night of his conversion and wrote, "This shows that the Lord may begin his work in different ways. For I have not the least doubt that on that evening He began a work of grace in me, though I obtained joy without any deep sorrow of heart, and with scarcely any knowledge. But that evening was the turning point in my life."[1]

God begins His work in each of us in different ways, but He longs to demonstrate His grace in mighty ways according to His purpose for our lives.

Has God ever supplied a need that you never mentioned to anyone, as He did for the orphans in George Müller's house? If so, what happened?

Have you ever felt God prompting you to meet a need that no one had told you about, as He did with the baker who brought bread for the orphans? If so, what happened?

_____

_____

_____

_____

What do you believe God is calling you to do? What are the needs involved with that calling?

_____

_____

_____

_____

Do you trust God to provide for them? What can cause you to doubt sometimes?

_____

_____

_____

_____

Dear Lord, help me trust that You will supply all that I need for the ministry You call me to do. Amen.

REFLECTION AND APPLICATION

Day 7

Dear Lord, help me be joyful in doing the work You have planned for me. Help me trust that You will supply my needs. Amen.

Not everyone is called to missionary work or to start a new ministry. The Lord wants us to be faithful in little ways, too.

Teresa and her husband led a small-group Bible study for singles in their home. When the study began, members agreed to take turns bringing refreshments for the group. As time went on, however, the hectic work schedules of the single men and women made it difficult for any of them to commit. Teresa agreed to provide treats every week.

It wasn't long before Teresa found herself grumbling about the all the money and time she spent on refreshments with so little thanks in return. When she realized how bitter she was becoming, she prayed for God's grace and peace.

The group had been studying various people in the Old Testament, and as Teresa thought about all they had learned, it occurred to her that she could make the weekly treats part of their learning experience if she investigated foods eaten in Bible times. She thanked the Lord for the idea and got to work.

Not only were her creative dishes a culinary hit with the group, but Teresa also looked forward with joy to researching and preparing each week's refreshment! And incredibly, as news spread about Teresa's delicious and educational delights, the number of people who came to study God's Word doubled in only a few weeks!

What has God impressed in your mind or heart to do lately?

_____

_____

_____

_____

_____

What do you *not* have peace about doing? Have you prayed for peace and grace?

_____

_____

_____

_____

Stephen's example in Acts showed us a man willing to serve God in any task, as well as someone ready to suffer for his faith. What small tasks are you doing that you can do for God (perhaps even cooking, mowing the yard or laundry)? How can you dedicate these tasks to His name?

_____

_____

_____

_____

_____

Dear Lord, thank You for Your grace and peace. Help me listen to
Your direction. Motivate me to act. Amen.

Note

1. J. Gilchrist Lawson, "George Frederick Müller," Christian Biography Resources. http://www.wholesomewords.org/biography/bmuller2.html (accessed May 2010).

Group Prayer Requests

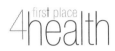

Today's Date: _____

Name	Request

Results

_____
_____
_____
_____
_____

sharing
grace

SCRIPTURE MEMORY VERSE

*Therefore go and make disciples of all nations . . .
teaching them to obey everything I have commanded you.
And surely I am with you always, to the very end of the age.*
MATTHEW 28:19-20

It's exciting to receive good news! We rejoice and then want to share. We may get on Facebook to let people know, phone friends and family, and tell our neighbors what has happened. The better the news, the more we want to share and celebrate. We may even party with family or friends.

God wants us to share the blessings we receive, especially the good news that Jesus died to bring salvation to anyone who believes. When we first hear and believe, we are excited. However, after a while our relationship with God can seem like "old news." We can become complacent and forget our excitement and the importance of telling others about Jesus. Yet each new blessing or answer to prayer we receive is an opportunity to thank God and tell others of His limitless grace.

This week's memory verse represents one of the last instructions Jesus gave before He ascended to heaven. Jesus told His disciples to teach others all that He had taught them. He commissioned them to share their faith. As followers of Christ, this commandment is for us, too. This week, we will explore how God's grace equips us to be ministers of the gospel.

Day 1

THE EXCITEMENT OF SHARING GOOD NEWS

Dear Father, help me rejoice in my blessings and share the good news with others. Amen.

God used four lepers to demonstrate the joy of sharing good news. It all began when the lepers thought that they had lost all hope. Read the story in 2 Kings 7:3-16. What did the lepers decide to do, and why (see verses 3-4)?

_____

_____

_____

_____

The lepers had so little hope that they chose to give themselves up rather than starve to death. But God had already prepared to meet their needs. Why did the soldiers flee the camp so fast that they took nothing with them (see verses 5-7)?

_____

_____

_____

_____

What did the lepers do when they found the Arameans' camp empty (see verse 8)?

_____

_____

_____

After they had eaten their fill, what did they say to each other (see verse 9)?

_____

_____

_____

_____

Good news is too good to keep to yourself! How does this story influence you to share the good news of your salvation?

_____

_____

_____

_____

What happened when the lepers shared their good news (see verses 10-16)?

_____

_____

_____

_____

Those with whom you share your good news may be skeptical at first. Some will accept quickly, while others will investigate and think things through. Today, pray for those with whom you will share the good news, asking that their hearts will be open to receiving God's grace.

Dear Father, thank You for all the blessings You send. Help me share the great joy I receive through Your grace. Amen.

EQUIPPED TO SHARE

Day 2

Dear Father, give me wisdom to share my faith and grace to know what to say. Amen.

The apostle Paul changed his life and focus once he encountered Jesus and became a believer. He accepted the responsibility to share his faith with Gentiles, even though he grew up as a devout Jew. Read Romans 15:14-19. What did Paul believe about believers (see verse 14)?

_____

_____

_____

_____

What was his goal in preaching to the Gentiles (see verse 16)?

_____

_____

_____

_____

Paul declared the competence of all believers to share their faith. His boldness in his own ministry, preaching to the Gentiles, came from God's grace. When God asks us to share our faith, we can do so in confidence that He sees us as fit and prepared to do it. Let's find out how Paul followed Christ's instruction to share his faith. Read Romans 15:17-19. To whom did Paul give the credit for the results of his ministry?

_____

_____

_____

_____

What did people experience from the Holy Spirit through Paul?

_____

_____

_____

_____

Paul spoke about what he had lived and experienced. He focused on his calling to preach, and the Holy Spirit worked to change hearts and show God's glory in miracles and signs. According to Romans 15:20-21, what goal did Paul have?

_____

_____

_____

Paul obeyed Christ's commandment given in this week's memory verse: "Therefore go and make disciples of all nations . . . teaching them to obey everything I have commanded you. And surely I am with you always, to the very end of the age" (Matthew 28:19-20). Read Acts 1:8 and John 14:16-17,26. What else did Jesus promise He would do? How would it help?

_____

_____

_____

_____

Imagine that you are talking with Paul about your reluctance to share the good news. What do you think he would tell you? What would he remind you about God's grace?

_____

_____

_____

_____

Dear Lord, give me the courage to share the gospel. Help me to trust
that the Holy Spirit will help me witness. Amen.

NETWORKING WITH GRACE

Day 3

Dear Lord, help me to learn from other Christians, to help when
I can and to share my faith. Amen.

We are connected to other Christians in love, fellowship and grace. Their examples encourage us to reach out to people who don't yet know Jesus. Let's look at how Christians are networked to work together to share the gospel by looking at what Paul wrote to the church at Colossae.

Read Colossians 1:1-8. What had Paul done since hearing of the people's faith?

_____

_____

_____

Who shared the gospel with these people? What was the result (see verse 8)?

_____

_____

_____

According to Colossians 1:6, what produces fruit? Where is the fruit produced?

_____

_____

_____

Paul was continuing to bring the gospel to other places even as the church in Colossae shared it with their neighbors. The fruit of the gospel was springing up all over! Read 1 Thessalonians 5:11. What are we to do for one another? How can this help us share the Good News with others?

_____

_____

_____

Look at Colossians 1:6 again. How has the grace of God had an impact on your life since you first heard about it?

_____

_____

_____

Our testimony—the changes that have occurred in us since our salvation—is the witness we can share with others about God's grace. Yet many people have fears about sharing their testimony. Read Luke 12:11-12. Who will help you know what to say when it is important to witness to others?

_____

_____

_____

_____

Witnessing is not a time to condemn others but an opportunity to share how God has changed you. Speak with gentleness and respect, and trust God's Holy Spirit to give you the words to say.

Dear Lord, I am thankful to be part of a large network of Christians. Give me the words I need to say to share my faith. Amen.

CALLING TO SHARE GOD'S GRACE

Day 4

Dear Lord, give me grace and strength to witness about You and my faith. Help me share the good news with joy. Amen.

We think of pastors and missionaries as people God has called to preach the gospel, but everyone is called to help spread the kingdom of God according to his or her gifts. God uses our gifts in many different ways and uses our story (or testimony) to help others see the difference God's grace can make. The way we live as believers also witnesses how God's grace changes us.

Read Matthew 5:14-16. What metaphor does Jesus use in these verses? What does He say you must do?

___

How can you let your light shine at home? At work? With your friends? At your gym?

___

According to Ecclesiastes 3:11, what has God put in the heart of every human being?

_____

_____

_____

Read Romans 1:20. How can those who don't yet trust Jesus see God at work around them?

_____

_____

_____

People may have a hard time admitting that they have sinned against God, and reject your message. What did Jesus say about rejection in Luke 10:16?

_____

_____

_____

We should view rejection when we share our faith as a rejection of God, not of ourselves. The apostles stayed focused on the goal, not the persecution. According to Acts 5:41-42, how did the apostles react to persecution?

_____

_____

_____

_____

The apostles had an unquenchable passion for sharing the good news of salvation through God's grace. Today, think of some reasons why you want to share your faith.

Dear Lord, I am thankful for Your grace and want to let others know how You have changed me. Give me the grace to witness. Amen.

ADMINISTERING GOD'S GRACE

Dear Lord, I want to serve You faithfully and share my faith. Help me to know Your purpose for me and to use my gifts to serve You. Amen.

Grace is not a one-time gift; it's a blessing we receive continually. Likewise, we should continually share God's grace with others. God has given each of us gifts that are to be used to build one another up. Let's look at how we can use our gifts to share our faith and minister with grace.

Read 1 Peter 4:9-11 and Romans 12:4-8. What spiritual gifts are found in these passages?

_____

_____

_____

_____

In the following table, list how each of these gifts can be used as a testimony of God's grace.

Gift	How it can be used as a testimony of God's grace
Hospitality	
Speaking	
Serving	
Prophesying	
Teaching	

Gift	How it can be used as a testimony of God's grace
Encouraging	
Giving	
Leading	
Showing mercy	

Do you know your spiritual gift? If not, ask your pastor or First Place 4 Health leader for some resources to identify it. If so, how are you using your gift as a testimony to God's grace?

_____

_____

_____

_____

_____

Dear Lord, thank You for Your great love for me. Help me to love others and share my gifts with them. Amen.

Day 6

REFLECTION AND APPLICATION

Dear Father, You are the one who gives grace and changes hearts. Help me serve You as I witness to others. Amen.

Chris wanted what he saw in his boss's life. He couldn't define it, but he knew the man had something different—something that gave him real joy and peace. He saw the same quality in the man's wife. Finally, after weeks of observation, Chris asked, "I see something different in you. What is it?"

His boss replied, "I'm a Christian, and it's Jesus Christ." That unexpected answer shook Chris a bit. He didn't want to become some freak and didn't think he needed God. He tuned out to whatever else his boss said.

A few years later, Chris had moved away. At his new job, he observed a co-worker who seemed to be such a great person and so loving. He wanted what that co-worker had, and finally asked him, "What makes you so loving?"

The man responded, "I'm a Christian and Jesus changed my heart and my life. He gives me the grace every day to love others." That overwhelmed Chris, because he didn't want to know Jesus or become religious. He continued with his own life and tried to ignore what his co-worker had said.

A few years later, Chris moved to another city. Once again, he encountered a boss he greatly admired, but this time he avoided asking the man about what made him different (Chris was pretty sure he already knew the answer).

Then Chris faced some major life problems and didn't know where to turn. Desperate, he decided that if his boss gave him the same answer as the two previous men, Chris would have to consider learning more about Jesus.

Yes, the man was a Christian—and, yes, the difference in his life was Jesus Christ. Chris started attending his boss's church, along with his wife, and it wasn't long before Jesus was making a difference in their lives, too.

Sharing your faith doesn't mean that someone will instantly want to listen or believe. You may be the first person, the third person or the tenth person to come along at just the right time, willing to give an answer for what you believe. The results are in God's hands. Your part is to persist in sharing and living your faith.

Who told you about Jesus?

_____

_____

_____

_____

Did you listen when you first heard about Jesus? Why or why not?

_____

_____

_____

_____

What made you want to become a Christian?

_____

_____

_____

_____

Consider your reasons for becoming a Christian and reflect on that before you share your faith again. Today, say a prayer for the person to whom you want to witness. Ask God to show you how to use your own experience coming to Him as you seek to share your faith.

> *Dear Lord, nudge me to speak out and share my faith.*
> *Help me to trust the results to You. Amen.*

Day 7 — REFLECTION AND APPLICATION

Dear Lord, I'm amazed to know how much grace You give.
Help me to share Your grace. Amen.

As we conclude this study, we will take a few moments today to review some Bible verses about God's grace. After reading each verse, write a brief statement about what the verse means for your life.

"I do not set aside the grace of God, for if righteousness could be gained through the law, Christ died for nothing" (Galatians 2:21).

_____

_____

_____

_____

_____

_____

"For all have sinned and fall short of the glory of God, and are justified freely by his grace through the redemption that came by Christ Jesus" (Romans 3:23-24).

_____

_____

_____

_____

_____

"Grow in the grace and knowledge of our Lord and Savior Jesus Christ" (2 Peter 3:18).

_____

_____

_____

_____

"Let your conversation be always full of grace, seasoned with salt, so that you may know how to answer everyone" (Colossians 4:6).

_____

_____

_____

_____

"God is able to make all grace abound to you, so that in all things at all times, having all that you need, you will abound in every good work" (2 Corinthians 9:8).

_____

_____

_____

_____

_____

"All this is for your benefit, so that the grace that is reaching more and more people may cause thanksgiving to overflow to the glory of God" (2 Corinthians 4:15).

_____

_____

_____

_____

_____

Dear Lord, thank You for Your Word, which reminds me of Your infinite grace. May I hide Your Word in my heart. Amen.

Group Prayer Requests

4 first place
health

Today's Date: _____

Name	Request

Results

_____
_____
_____
_____
_____

time to celebrate!

To help shape your brief victory celebration testimony, work through the following questions in your prayer journal:

Day One: List some of the benefits you have gained by allowing the Lord to transform your life through this 12-week First Place 4 Health session. Be sure to list benefits you have received in the physical, mental, emotional and spiritual realms of your being.

Day Two: In what ways have you most significantly changed *mentally*? Have you seen a shift in the ways you think about yourself, food, your relationships or God? How has Scripture memory been a part of these shifts?

Day Three: In what ways have you most significantly changed *emotionally*? Have you begun to identify how your feelings influence your relationship to food and exercise? What are you doing to stay aware of your emotions, both positive and negative?

Day Four: In what ways have you most significantly changed *spiritually*? How has your relationship with God deepened? How has drawing closer to Him made a difference in the other three areas of your life?

Day Five: In what ways have you most significantly changed *physically*? Have you met or exceeded your weight/measurement goals? How has your health improved the past 12 weeks?

Day Six: Was there one person in your First Place 4 Health group who was particularly encouraging to you? How did their kindness make a difference in your First Place 4 Health journey?

Day Seven: Summarize the previous six questions into a one-page testimony, or "faith story," to share at your group's victory celebration.

May our gracious Lord bless and keep you as you continue to keep Him first in all things!

Walking in Grace
leader discussion guide

For in-depth information, guidance and helpful tips about leading a successful First Place 4 Health group, study the *First Place 4 Health Leader's Guide*. In it, you will find valuable answers to most of your questions, as well as personal insights from many First Place 4 Health group leaders.

For the group meetings in this session, be sure to read and consider each week's discussion topics several days before the meeting—some questions and activities require supplies and/or planning to complete. Also, if you are leading a large group, plan to break into smaller groups for discussion and then come together as a large group to share your answers and responses. Make sure to appoint a capable leader for each small group so that discussions stay focused and on track (and be sure each group records their answers!).

week one: welcome to *walking in grace*

During this first week, welcome the members to your group, provide a brief overview of the First Place 4 Health program, explain what is expected of the participants at each of the weekly meetings, and collect the Member Surveys. (See the *First Place 4 Health Leader's Guide* for a detailed outline of how to conduct the first week's meeting.)

week two: gift of grace

Begin today's session by asking the participants in your group to describe the images the words "gift" and "grace" bring to their minds.

Talk to your group about the apostle Paul, who began his adult life as an enemy of Christians. Ask what people know about him (remember that some members may have little Bible knowledge) and share his conversion story, found in Acts 9.

Lead a discussion on how change happens. There are two main catalysts for change. One is to reach a point where a person thinks, *I can't go on like this anymore.* The other is when a person envisions how life could be and how a change will make life better. Talk about how God's Word gives us forgiveness and freedom from the past and vision and hope for a better life.

Ask members to describe how, with God's grace, they have been able to follow the First Place 4 Health program and how it is changing them. Discuss the excitement of positive changes.

Discuss the week's memory verse, 2 Corinthians 3:17. Be sure to allow plenty of time to talk about how God gives us freedom to follow Him rather than coercing us. Discuss why choosing to join First Place 4 Health has been a good decision.

Talk about how God's grace helped people get through difficulties. Review the verses studied in Philippians 4:4-6, Romans 12:1-3 and Titus 2:12. Ask members what these verses mean to them. Discuss how with the grace of God we renew our minds, learn to live more sensibly and endure with steadfastness.

Ask each member to briefly summarize his or her hopes for change, and how he or she needs God's grace to make those changes. End today's lesson by reading 1 Peter 1:13-16 as your prayer for the group.

week three: grace to be ourselves

Ask participants to talk about how God created us and understands our thoughts and desires. How do the members feel about God knowing them even before they were born? What does it mean to them to be handcrafted by God?

Read Proverbs 3:5-6. Talk about how setting aside time for Bible study and prayer is an important way to put God first. How is this going for the members? Is anyone frustrated by his or her lack of time or motivation?

Proverbs 4:7-13 lists the many benefits of wisdom. On a whiteboard or flipchart, make two columns. For the first column, ask members to list the wisdom they have learned this week from Bible study and First Place 4 Health. In the second column, ask them to brainstorm the benefits of that wisdom.

Review 1 Peter 5:10. Ask members to think about how "suffering for a little while" might be an important part of the process of restoration. How might this relate to daily exercise, avoiding high-calorie foods and dealing with the underlying emotional issues of chronic over-eating?

Talk about how a person needs rest and how that fits with living a healthy and balanced life. Who is struggling with getting enough rest? What do they need to change in order to get enough?

This week's study also looked at Daniel and his friends' choice to eat healthy. As members have followed the Live It Plan this week, what have they noticed about how their bodies feel? Do they have more energy? Less? Is it easier or more difficult to focus on tasks?

Let members share the compliments they have written for other members of the group. Talk about the importance of encouraging one another, and then close in prayer.

week four: saved by grace

Before the meeting, ask a couple of volunteers to share how they came to know Christ (their testimonies). Let them know they should share for 2 to 3 minutes. After you open the meeting, invite these volunteers to share their testimonies.

There was some scientific information given throughout the week's study about the miracle of blood. What characteristic of human blood made the biggest impression on members' minds as a metaphor for the spiritual life?

In the book of Nehemiah, the broken wall of Jerusalem is a "symptom" of the people's hidden sin. Ask members to think about what outward symptoms in their life indicate inward sin. Open the door to conversation by sharing your own answer. (*Note:* It is important to emphasize that being overweight is *not* in itself a sin, but it can be a symptom of putting food before God, self-hatred or other sins.)

On Day 4, the members read about plans and works that God has prepared for us. He wants us to prosper and to partner with Him. Ask participants to share any plans they believe God has prepared for them.

It's as hard for us to comprehend heaven as it is for a developing baby to understand life outside the womb. Discuss the glimpses of heaven in the Bible and the joy of knowing our future is in heaven.

God's grace transformed both the apostle Paul and John Newton from selfish sinners to generous believers. Is anyone in the group troubled by their sinful past? Let them know that God forgives completely by His grace, and opens wide the door to a new future with Him.

Review Ephesians 4:1. On Day 7, we discussed how the Greek word translated "worthy" in this verse can be understood both as "balanced" and "becoming." As we balance the knowledge of our calling with action, we become the people God created us to be. How are members learning to balance what they are learning with action?

Close the meeting in prayer, asking God to bless the members' efforts with His grace.

week five: encouragement of grace

Discuss some of the encouraging and kind words participants received this week. How did the words make them feel? How were they inspired and motivated?

The Good Samaritan went out of his way to help a stranger. Let members share when a stranger helped them or when they helped a stranger.

On Day Three, the group looked at how words begin in our hearts. Why does this make morning prayer or devotions so important? Discuss what to do when we notice our speech is filled with anger, envy or other negative emotions.

Encouragement unites people and builds team spirit. Ask members to share how encouragement helps them feel part of a team.

On Day Five, the group studied praise as a fruit of our lips. Talk about how praise changes our perspective as we reflect on God's ability and promises. Ask participants to share praises.

Writing letters is becoming a lost art, yet a written note of encouragement can really make a big difference. Pass out note cards and pens and invite members to take 10 minutes on their own to write a note of encouragement to another member. Collect all the envelopes and mail them to their recipients sometime during the week. (Make sure you have everyone's address!)

Emphasize that encouragement is one of the most important aspects of First Place 4 Health. Ask for volunteers to share about a time when encouragement from another member helped them stay on track with the Live It Plan.

Recite the memory verse (Hebrews 3:12-13) together, and then close in prayer.

week six: transformed by grace

On Day Two, the members read how Jesus felt compassion for hungry people and gave them an abundant feast. How is God giving the group abundant grace and supplying their mental, emotional, spiritual and physical needs?

Share from your own life about when you have sowed seeds that reaped a harvest you did not want (e.g., you sowed over-eating and reaped being overweight, or you sowed angry words and reaped a broken relationship). What seeds have other members sown and then regretted the harvest they reaped?

In order to reap a harvest that pleases God, we must plant the right seeds, nurture them as they grow and wait on His grace to bring them to maturity. What seeds have members planted for the harvest they *want* to reap? What are they doing to nurture that crop in their lives? How do they see God's grace at work to bring the harvest He has planned for them?

Jesus is an extravagant giver, especially when it comes to love and grace. Ask members to share a time they have seen Him bless beyond what they had expected or imagined. Briefly review Mary's story on Day Six. Ask participants to share a time they unexpectedly received more than they gave.

Grace, like water, has many benefits. Review some of water's miraculous properties and ask members to describe which aspects of grace are most important to them right now.

Recite the memory verse together (Romans 3:22-24), and then close in prayer.

week seven: connected to grace

Being connected to Jesus, the Vine, gives us grace and a ready supply of help. It also connects us to other Christians. Ask members how being connected to their First Place 4 Health group has changed their perspective on what it means to be connected to the Body of Christ.

Pruning doesn't sound like fun, but it aids growth. How have members been pruned in the past by the Master Gardener? What fruit did their lives bear because of His pruning? How are members being pruned right now?

Early Christians eagerly studied God's Word and became united in purpose and love. Their enthusiasm and excitement encouraged growth. Ask the members if they feel a similar enthusiasm when it comes to studying God's Word. If not, is something standing in their way? (Be sure not to be judgmental as people share where they are at; just accept and encourage them.)

Ask for a volunteer to read Ephesians 1:2-9 and discuss the passage, verse by verse. What are the spiritual blessings listed here? What do they mean for our lives?

Review the Beatitudes given by Jesus in His Sermon on the Mount (Matthew 5:3-10). Discuss how these promises can help us endure trials in the here and now.

On Days Five and Six, members were introduced to the P-R-A-Y-E-R acrostic. Ask if anyone tried this method of prayer this week? If so, what were the results?

Close the meeting in prayer, using the P-R-A-Y-E-R acrostic. Ask for one volunteer to pray about each element.

week eight: strengthened by grace

This week's memory verse states that God is a strong tower. Ask members to share a time when they ran to God for safety. What danger or problem were they facing? How did God keep them safe?

On Day Three, the group looked at the importance of trusting God instead of wealth or pride. Have a volunteer read Matthew 6:19-20, and then ask members to brainstorm how to store up treasures in heaven.

On Day Three, the members also looked at the instruction in 1 Timothy 6:17-19 to be rich in good deeds and be generous with our wealth. What are some ways that the group can pool their resources and share resources with those in need? Come up with a list of ways to share your wealth, and then plan to do so.

The image of God as a tower is also used in Scripture to describe His provision for us. Discuss how God is providing for members' needs out of His storehouse of blessing.

Ask members to discuss how truly believing that God will provide enough can help them avoid overeating. Does anyone sometimes overeat out of fear or anxiety? How can trusting God give us strength to make good eating choices?

On Day Four, the members looked at some of the connections between strength, courage and joy. Ask if anyone has known a person who was able to remain joyful even during tough times. How can that person's example inspire us to stay strong during trials?

Close in prayer, thanking God for the strength of His grace and praying for each member by name.

week nine: living in grace

Begin the meeting by asking each member to share one thing for which they are thankful. Once everyone has shared, review some of the benefits from this week's introduction of being thankful.

Have two volunteers read Luke 7:36-50. Ask members to put themselves in the room with Jesus, the sinful woman and Simon the Pharisee. With whom would they most identify? Knowing that they have been forgiven completely through God's grace, how do members want to respond to Jesus? (Answers may be a simple as "give thanks in prayer," but encourage everyone to think outside the box.)

On Day Two, the members examined how Hannah poured out her heart to God. She didn't try to put on a smile and act like her life was fine. Ask members to share how being open and honest about their struggles opens the door to God's grace.

Both Hannah and David did unexpected things to express their thanks. David took his best friend's son, Mephibosheth, into his own home even though he had a claim to David's throne. How can being grateful help us to act in ways that honor God above ourselves?

David wrote many psalms expressing gratitude to God, even when he was in his darkest hours. Review Psalms 27, 28 and 31. Which verses or passages were most meaningful to members this week? Ask if anyone wants to share the psalm they wrote on Day Five.

Discuss the importance of journaling. Whether it is a personal journal, a prayer journal, a thankfulness journal or a diary to track answers to prayer, making a practice of writing down your journey with God is a spiritual discipline that will bear fruit. Who in the group is keeping a journal? How is it having an impact on their journey?

For the closing prayer, ask each member to offer a one-sentence prayer of thanks.

week ten: responding in grace

This week's study was all about success stories from the Bible. Ask members which story was most inspiring to them and why.

When Esther made the decision to go to the king, she asked her people to fast and pray on her behalf. How has prayer prepared the members to act with grace? When was the last time the members requested prayer from others?

Paul and Barnabas shared the results of their missionary trip with the people who had prayed for them. Ask members to share an answer to group prayer they have received. What has the group been praying for? How is God answering those prayers?

Stephen is an amazing example of a humble man who did both small and great tasks for the Lord. What "small" tasks are members trying to do to God's glory? How is that changing their perspective of those tasks?

Esther, Paul, Barnabas and Stephen were all called upon to step out in faith, without knowing the outcome. Ask if anyone in the group is feeling called to step out in faith. Take a few minutes to pray for those members, bless them and ask God for His guidance and protection over them.

Grace and peace are connected in many of the verses we have studied. Ask members how God's grace has given them peace to face their circumstances. How has God's peace made a difference on their First Place 4 Health journey?

On a whiteboard or flipchart, list some of the group members' gifts in one column. In the other, brainstorm ways those gifts can benefit the whole group. To close the meeting, read Romans 8:28 aloud together as a reminder and a benediction.

week eleven: sharing grace

This week's verse is from the Great Commission. Recite Matthew 28:19-20 together, and then ask for one or two volunteers to share how they first heard the good news. Who shared God's grace with him or her? What was it that he or she saw in that person that made them want to know Christ?

Review the story from Day One. Point out that in ancient times, lepers were outcasts from society. However, that didn't keep these four lepers from sharing the good news. Discuss if any members have felt that their weight or other problems keep them from sharing their faith.

Ask them to imagine how God can use those weaknesses for His glory. How might He use their struggles to draw others close to Him?

Paul believed every Christian is competent and equipped to share their faith. From your own experience, share how you have sometimes *not* felt competent or equipped. In what ways are you insecure? Open the floor for others to share their insecurities about witnessing.

When people reject the message of God's grace, it can sometimes feel that they are rejecting *us*. Discuss how this fear of rejection plays into our reluctance to share our testimony. How can we overcome this fear?

Last week, we discussed how each member's gifts could benefit the whole group. This week, use a whiteboard or flipchart to list how these gifts can point unbelievers to God's grace. How can God use our spiritual gifts to draw people to Him?

Day Seven gave the members an opportunity to review some of the many Scriptures that talk about God's grace. Ask members to share which verse is the most meaningful to them and why.

As a closing prayer, have everyone read 2 Thessalonians 2:16 together as a benediction and a blessing on one another.

week twelve: time to celebrate!

Even though most of your meeting this week will be a victory celebration, take some time at the beginning of the meeting to talk about how much God loves each person in the group and how each of us is called to love our brothers and sisters in Christ. (See "Planning a Victory Celebration" in the *First Place 4 Health Leader's Guide* for ideas about throwing a successful celebration for your group.)

For the rest of the study time, allow each member to tell his or her Walking in Grace story. Give members an equal opportunity to share the goals they set for themselves at the beginning of the session and talk about the challenges and good things God has done for them throughout the process. Don't allow the more talkative group members to monopolize all the time. Even the quiet members need an opportunity to share their stories and successes! Even those who have not met their goals have still been part of the journey, so allow them to share and talk about why they did not succeed.

Making a commitment to continue in First Place 4 Health is an important part of victory. Be sure to talk about your group's future plans, and make each person feel welcome to continue to journey with you. To end the discussion session, have everyone read 2 Corinthians 3:14 aloud together as a benediction and a blessing to each other.

First Place 4 Health menu plans

Each menu plan is based on approximately 1,400 to 1,500 calories per day. All recipe and menu exchanges were determined using the Master-Cook software, a program that accesses a database containing more than 6,000 food items prepared using the United States Department of Agriculture (USDA) publications and information from food manufacturers. As with any nutritional program, MasterCook calculates the nutritional values of the recipes based on ingredients. Nutrition may vary due to how the food is prepared, where the food comes from, soil content, season, ripeness, processing and method of preparation. For these reasons, please use the recipes and menu plans as approximate guides. Consult a physician and/or a registered dietitian before starting a weight-loss program.

For those who need more calories, add the following to the 1,400-calorie plan:

- 1,800 calories: 2 ounce equivalent of meat, 3 ounce equivalent of bread, $^1/_2$ cup vegetable serving, 1 tsp. fat

- 2,000 calories: 2 ounce equivalent of meat, 4 ounce equivalent of bread, $^1/_2$ cup vegetable serving, 3 tsp. fat

- 2,200 calories: 2 ounce equivalent of meat, 5 ounce equivalent of bread, $^1/_2$ cup vegetable serving, $^1/_2$ cup fruit serving, 5 tsp. fat

- 2,400 calories: 2 ounce equivalent of meat, 6 ounce equivalent of bread, 1 cup vegetable serving, $^1/_2$ cup fruit serving, 6 tsp. fat

First Week Grocery List

Produce
- [ ] apple
- [ ] bananas
- [ ] blueberries
- [ ] broccoli
- [ ] cabbage with carrots slaw mix (1 pkg.)
- [ ] cantaloupe
- [ ] carrots
- [ ] cauliflower
- [ ] garlic
- [ ] grape tomatoes
- [ ] green bell pepper
- [ ] green onion
- [ ] mushrooms
- [ ] onion
- [ ] potatoes
- [ ] raspberries
- [ ] red bell pepper
- [ ] red onion
- [ ] romaine lettuce
- [ ] small red potatoes
- [ ] yellow squash
- [ ] zucchini

Baking/Cooking Products
- [ ] all-fruit spread, apricot
- [ ] applesauce, unsweetened
- [ ] basil, dried
- [ ] basil pesto
- [ ] brown rice
- [ ] Dijon mustard
- [ ] dill, dried
- [ ] dried cranberries
- [ ] five-spice powder
- [ ] French onion dip
- [ ] hollandaise sauce
- [ ] marinara sauce
- [ ] nonstick cooking spray
- [ ] olive oil
- [ ] pepper
- [ ] pimientos
- [ ] rosemary
- [ ] salad dressing, light Italian
- [ ] salad dressing, lowfat buttermilk Ranch
- [ ] salsa
- [ ] salt
- [ ] soy sauce
- [ ] Splenda®
- [ ] stuffing mix, herb-seasoned
- [ ] sugar
- [ ] sweet and sour sauce
- [ ] syrup, light
- [ ] vanilla extract
- [ ] Wish-Bone Citrus Splash Vinaigrette Salad Dressing®

Breads and Cereals
- [ ] bowtie pasta
- [ ] breadsticks
- [ ] cinnamon-raisin bread
- [ ] cornflakes
- [ ] dinner rolls, whole-grain
- [ ] French bread
- [ ] Grape Nuts® cereal
- [ ] puffed rice cereal
- [ ] ramen noodles, chicken flavored
- [ ] saltine crackers
- [ ] sourdough bread

Canned Foods

- ❏ beef consommé
- ❏ chicken broth, reduced-sodium
- ❏ Dole® tropical fruit cocktail in passion fruit juice
- ❏ Mandarin orange sections
- ❏ petite-diced tomatoes with green pepper and onion
- ❏ pineapple chunks in juice

Dairy Products

- ❏ cheddar cheese (2%)
- ❏ cream cheese, light with chives and onion
- ❏ half and half, fat-free
- ❏ margarine, light
- ❏ Mexican-blend cheese, reduced-fat
- ❏ milk, nonfat
- ❏ nonfat yogurt, artificially sweetened pineapple-flavored
- ❏ nonfat yogurt, artificially sweetened vanilla-flavored
- ❏ Parmesan cheese
- ❏ sour cream, light
- ❏ whipping cream

Juices

- ❏ orange juice

Frozen Foods

- ❏ asparagus
- ❏ California-style vegetables
- ❏ cornbread twists (1 pkg.)
- ❏ Italian-cut green beans
- ❏ oriental stir-fry vegetables
- ❏ waffles

Meat and Poultry

- ❏ beef tenderloin steaks
- ❏ chicken breasts, boneless, skinless
- ❏ chicken thighs, boneless, skinless
- ❏ eggs
- ❏ ground beef, extra lean

First Week Meals and Recipes

DAY 1

Breakfast

½ medium cantaloupe, topped with
   1 cup artificially sweetened pineapple-flavored nonfat yogurt and
   ¼ cup Grape Nuts® cereal

Nutritional Information: 183 calories; 1g fat (4.2% calories from fat); 12g protein; 34g carbohydrate; 3g dietary fiber; 3mg cholesterol; 153mg sodium.

Lunch

Quick and Crunchy Chicken Salad

8 oz. diced cooked chicken breast
1 16-oz. pkg. shredded cabbage with
   carrots slaw mix
¼ cup sliced red onion
1 3-oz. pkg. ramen noodles, crumbled
½ cup bottled Wish-Bone Citrus
   Splash Vinaigrette Salad Dressing®
1 15-oz. Mandarin orange sections,
   drained
4 cups chopped romaine lettuce

Combine chicken, slaw mix and red onion in a large bowl. Add crumbled ramen (save the seasoning packet for another use). Pour dressing over the top and toss well to coat. Gently stir in Mandarin orange sections. Spoon equal amounts onto each of four 1-cup servings of chopped lettuce. Serve each with 1-ounce breadstick. Serves 4.

Nutritional Information: 516 calories; 22g fat (37.5% calories from fat); 26g protein; 55g carbohydrate; 5g dietary fiber; 48mg cholesterol; 620mg sodium.

Dinner

Steak with Mushroom Sauce

2 2"-thick beef tenderloin steaks
   (about 1 lb. total), trimmed of fat
salt and pepper
1 tsp. olive oil
8 oz. mushrooms, sliced
¼ cup beef consommé
¼ cup whipping cream
2 tsp. Dijon mustard

Season steaks with salt and pepper on both sides and set aside. Preheat olive oil in a large skillet over medium heat, and then add steaks and cook to desired doneness, turning once (about 10 minutes total for medium-rare and 14 minutes for medium). Transfer steaks to warm platter. Use same skillet to cook mushrooms 4 minutes over medium heat. Stir in consommé, cream and mustard. Cook and stir over medium heat 2 to 3 minutes or until slightly thickened. Add more seasoning to taste, if desired. Slice each steak into 6 pieces and place 3 pieces on each of 4 plates. Top each with 2 tablespoons mushroom sauce. Serve with 1 *Twice Baked Broccoli Potato* and a 1-ounce dinner roll. Serves 4.

Nutritional Information: 610 calories; 38g fat (54.9% calories from fat); 30g protein; 40g carbohydrate; 6g dietary fiber; 104mg cholesterol; 392mg sodium.

Twice-Baked Broccoli Potatoes

2 medium-sized baking potatoes
2 cups frozen broccoli florets
1 tbsp. light sour cream

1 tbsp. light margarine
salt and pepper
1 tbsp. shredded 2% cheddar
  cheese

Wash potatoes and prick skin several times with fork. Place the potatoes in microwave-safe dish and microwave on high for 5 minutes. Turn the potatoes over and cook for 4 minutes. Let sit for 2 minutes, and then slice in half lengthwise. Scoop out the pulp (being careful not to tear the surrounding skin) into medium bowl. Add broccoli, sour cream, margarine and salt and pepper. Mix well and refill skins with pulp mixture. Top with cheese and microwave for 2 to 3 minutes. Serves 4.

Nutritional Information: 124 calories; 3g fat (17.4% calories from fat); 5g protein; 22g carbohydrate; 4g dietary fiber; 3mg cholesterol; 71mg sodium.

DAY 2

Breakfast

1 cup puffed-rice cereal
½ medium banana
1 cup nonfat milk

Nutritional Information: 194 calories; 1g fat (3.6% calories from fat); 10g protein; 38g carbohydrate; 2g dietary fiber; 4mg cholesterol; 127mg sodium.

Lunch

Taco Pizza

½ lb. extra-lean ground beef
1 medium green bell pepper, diced
1 medium red onion, diced
½ cup prepared salsa (any kind)

1 11.5-oz. pkg. refrigerated cornbread twists
1 cup shredded reduced-fat Mexican-blend cheese

Preheat oven to 400° F. In medium nonstick skillet, cook ground beef, bell pepper and onion over medium heat until meat is browned. Drain and set aside. Unroll cornbread-twist dough—*but don't separate into strips*. Press dough onto the bottom of a 12″ round pizza pan. Spread salsa evenly over dough, sprinkle with meat mixture, and then top with cheese. Bake for 20 minutes or until crust is browned. Cut into 8 slices. Serve with ½ cup Dole® tropical fruit cocktail in passion-fruit juice. Serves 4.

Nutritional Information: 555 calories; 22g fat (35.5% calories from fat); 24g protein; 65g carbohydrate; 7g dietary fiber; 47mg cholesterol; 1,258mg sodium.

Dinner

Cranberry-Apricot Stuffed Chicken Breasts

4 boneless, skinless chicken breasts (about 1 lb.)
1½ cups herb-seasoned stuffing mix
½ cup apricot all-fruit spread, divided

½ cup dried cranberries, divided
¼ cup light margarine, melted, divided
nonstick cooking spray

Preheat oven to 400° F. Place each chicken breast between 2 pieces of plastic wrap, and then pound lightly until breasts are about ¼″ thick. Discard plastic and set chicken aside. In medium bowl, combine stuffing mix, ¼ cup cranberries, $1/3$ cup apricot spread and 3 tablespoons margarine. Stir until moistened and then set aside. Combine the remaining cranberries, apricot spread and margarine in small bowl, and then stir well and set aside. Divide the stuffing mixture evenly among the four breasts. Fold the sides of each breast over the stuffing and roll up, securing with a toothpick. Place stuffed breasts in a 3-quart baking dish coated with nonstick cooking spray, and then bake uncovered for 15 minutes. Remove the breasts from the oven and brush cranberry-apricot glaze mixture over the top of each. Bake 10 to 12 minutes more. Serve each breast with 1 serving *Veggie Mash* and 1 whole-grain dinner roll. Serves 4.

Nutritional Information: 509 calories; 15g fat (27.3% calories from fat); 34g protein; 58g carbohydrate; 6g dietary fiber; 71mg cholesterol; 874mg sodium.

Veggie Mash

3 cups sliced carrots (peel before slicing)
2 cups coarsely chopped cauliflower
1 cup coarsely chopped broccoli
½ 8-oz. container prepared French onion dip
½ tsp. black pepper

Place carrots in large saucepan, and then add water to cover. Bring to a boil and cook for 10 minutes. Add cauliflower and broccoli and cook 3 minutes more. Drain and coarsely mash the vegetables, and then stir in onion dip and black pepper. Serve warm. Serves 4.

Nutritional Information: 124 calories; 6g fat (42.1% calories from fat); 4g protein; 15g carbohydrate; 5g dietary fiber; 5mg cholesterol; 210mg sodium.

DAY 3

Breakfast

Turkey Bacon, Potato and Egg Scramble

2 slices turkey bacon, crisply cooked and crumbled
$1/_3$ lb. small red potatoes (about 2 potatoes), cubed
2 medium eggs, slightly beaten (or ½ cup egg substitute)
1 cup water
2 tbsp. nonfat milk
dash of salt and pepper
2 tsp. light margarine
2 tsp. sliced green onions
1 tsp. diced pimientos

Bring water and potatoes to a boil in a small saucepan. Let the potatoes cook 6 to 8 minutes or until tender, and then drain and set aside. In a small bowl, beat together eggs (or egg substitute), milk, salt and pepper with fork, and then set aside. Preheat a medium skillet over medium-high heat and add margarine. Sauté potatoes 3 to 4 minutes until slightly browned, and then add green onions and pimientos. Cook 1 minute more, stirring constantly. Pour the egg mixture over the potato mixture. As the mixture begins to set, gently stir until the uncooked eggs begin to cook and set. Cook 2 to

3 minutes or until the eggs are cooked but moist. Sprinkle with crumbled bacon and serve. Serve with 1 small banana and 1 6-ounce container of artificially sweetened nonfat yogurt (any flavor). Serves 2.

Nutritional Information: 377 calories; 10g fat (22.9% calories from fat); 18g protein; 57g carbohydrate; 5g dietary fiber; 202mg cholesterol; 402mg sodium.

Lunch

1 serving Long John Silver's® flavor-baked fish sandwich (no sauce)
side of green beans
side salad topped with
2 tbsp. lowfat dressing and
1 small orange

Nutritional Information: 604 calories; 25g fat (36.6% calories from fat); 22g protein; 76g carbohydrate; 10g dietary fiber; 47mg cholesterol; 1,494mg sodium.

Dinner

Pork Chops Dijon

4 1"-thick boneless pork loin chops (about 1 lb.), trimmed of fat
3 tbsp. Dijon mustard
2 tbsp. light Italian salad dressing
¼ tsp. black pepper
1 medium onion, halved and sliced
nonstick cooking spray

Combine mustard, salad dressing and pepper in a small bowl, and then mix well and set aside. Preheat a nonstick skillet coated with nonstick cooking spray over medium heat. Add chops to the skillet and cook for 2 minutes on each side. Remove chops from the skillet and set aside. In the same skillet, cook onion over medium heat for 2 to 3 minutes. Push onion to side of skillet and return chops to pan. Spread the mustard mixture over the chops, cover skillet and cook over medium-low heat for 15 minutes or until meat juices run clear. Spoon onion slices over the chops to serve. Serve with 1 serving *Vegetable Rice Pilaf* and 1 cup salad made with dark greens and 2 tablespoons light salad dressing. Serves 4.

Nutritional Information: 225 calories; 7g fat (37.4% calories from fat); 21g protein; 5g carbohydrate; 1g dietary fiber; 51mg cholesterol; 304mg sodium.

Vegetable Rice Pilaf

1 cup frozen mixed onion, celery and bell pepper
2 tbsp. light margarine
1 cup brown rice

4 cups reduced-sodium chicken
broth

2 cups frozen California-style
vegetables, chopped

In a large saucepan, sauté the onion blend in margarine over medium heat until tender. Add rice and cook until the rice is lightly browned. Carefully stir in chicken broth and bring the mixture to a boil. Reduce heat and simmer, covered, for 40 minutes. Stir in chopped vegetables and continue simmering for 5 minutes more, or until rice is tender and liquid is absorbed. Serves 4.

Nutritional Information: 323 calories; 6g fat (16.8% calories from fat); 13g protein; 55g carbohydrate; 6g dietary fiber; 0mg cholesterol; 898mg sodium.

DAY 4

Breakfast
2 slices light sourdough toast
1 tsp. light margarine

¾ cup blueberries
1 cup nonfat milk

Nutritional Information: 300 calories; 4g fat (12.4% calories from fat); 13g protein; 53g carbohydrate; 4g dietary fiber; 4mg cholesterol; 483mg sodium.

Lunch

Turkey-Sausage Noodle Soup
8 oz. cooked smoked turkey sausage,
thinly sliced
4 cups water
1 14.5-oz. can petite-diced tomatoes
with green pepper and onion

1 medium red bell pepper, cut into
½" squares
2 3-oz. pkgs. chicken-flavored ramen
noodles, crumbled
black pepper

Combine sausage, water, tomatoes (with liquid), bell pepper and ramen seasoning packets in a large saucepan. Bring to boil. Add noodles and return to boil for 2 to 3 minutes or until the noodles are tender. Add pepper to taste. Serve each with 1 cup carrot sticks and 1 small apple. Serves 4.

Nutritional Information: 544 calories; 20g fat (32.1% calories from fat); 15g protein; 80g carbohydrate; 11g dietary fiber; 40mg cholesterol; 1,348mg sodium.

Dinner

Italian Grilled Chicken
4 boneless, skinless chicken breasts (about 1 lb.)
¾ cup light Italian salad dressing

Place chicken breasts and dressing in a large sealable plastic bag. Refrigerate for 3 hours or overnight. When ready to use, remove the breasts from the dressing and grill over medium heat for 8 minutes, and then turn and grill for 4 to 5 minutes more or until chicken is no longer pink. Serve with 1 serving *Grilled Vegetable Kabobs* and 1 serving *Garlic Mashed Potatoes*. Serves 4.

Nutritional Information: 416 calories; 10g fat (21.6% calories from fat); 33g protein; 50g carbohydrate; 8g dietary fiber; 69mg cholesterol; 773mg sodium.

Grilled Vegetable Kabobs

5 12" to 14" wooden skewers
12 grape tomatoes
1 medium yellow squash, cut into
   1" pieces
1 medium zucchini, cut into
   1" pieces

1 red onion, cut into 1" pieces
1 medium red bell pepper,
   cut into 1" pieces
¼ cup light Italian salad dressing
salt and pepper

Thread all tomatoes onto 1 skewer and set aside. Thread the vegetable pieces onto the remaining skewers, alternating and using an equal amount of each vegetable on each skewer. Drizzle salad dressing over all skewers and season with salt and pepper. Grill mixed-vegetable kabobs over medium heat for 5 to 6 minutes or until tender, turning once. During the last 2 to 3 minutes, add tomato kabob to grill. Serves 4.

Nutritional Information: 130 calories; 3g fat (17.7% calories from fat); 5g protein; 26g carbohydrate; 7g dietary fiber; 1mg cholesterol; 155mg sodium.

Garlic Mashed Potatoes

3 cups peeled and cubed baking
   potatoes
1 to 2 tsp. chopped garlic
¼ cup fat-free half-and-half
1 tbsp. light margarine

¼ tsp. salt
dash of pepper

Place potatoes and garlic in a large saucepan, cover with water and bring to a boil. Reduce heat and simmer for 20 minutes. Drain and return to pan. Add half-and-half, margarine, salt and pepper to taste. To beat potato mixture, use electric mixer set on medium speed. Serves 4.

Nutritional Information: 114 calories; 2g fat (12.1% calories from fat); 2g protein; 22g carbohydrate; 2g dietary fiber; 0mg cholesterol; 190mg sodium.

DAY 5

Breakfast

Cinnamon French Toast

4 slices cinnamon-raisin bread
2 eggs, beaten
$^1/_3$ cup nonfat milk
1 tsp. sugar

¼ tsp. vanilla extract
1 tbsp. light syrup
nonstick cooking spray

Combine eggs, milk, sugar and vanilla in shallow dish, and then stir well and set aside. Preheat a nonstick skillet coated with nonstick cooking spray over medium heat. Dip bread slices into the egg mixture, turning to coat both sides. Cook for 3 to 4 minutes on each side or until the toast is golden brown. Drizzle each with 1½ teaspoons syrup and serve immediately. Serve with ½ cup fresh fruit and 1 cup nonfat milk. Serves 2.

Nutritional Information: 401 calories; 6g fat (13.6% calories from fat); 21g protein; 63g carbohydrate; 2g dietary fiber; 192mg cholesterol; 404mg sodium.

Lunch

1 cup Chick-fil-A Hearty Breast of
   Chicken Soup®
4 saltine crackers

1 small side carrot salad
1 small Chick-fil-A Icedream®
   cone

Nutritional Information: 605 calories; 21g fat (33.2% calories from fat); 1g protein; 93g carbohydrate; 6g dietary fiber; 45mg cholesterol; 1,530mg sodium.

Dinner

Sweet and Sour Chicken with Asian-Style Veggies

8 boneless, skinless chicken thighs
   (about 1 lb.)
2 tsp. olive oil
1 tsp. five-spice powder, divided
   (optional)
½ cup prepared sweet-and-sour
   sauce, divided

1 16-oz. pkg. frozen Oriental stir-fry
   vegetables
1 8-oz. can pineapple chunks in juice,
   drained
2 tsp. soy sauce
2 cups cooked brown rice

Preheat oven to 400° F. Arrange chicken thighs in the bottom of a 3-quart baking dish. Brush thighs with olive oil and sprinkle with ½ teaspoon five-spice powder. Bake, uncovered, for 20 minutes. While the chicken is cooking, combine the remaining five-spice powder, ¼ cup sweet-and-sour sauce, vegetables, pineapple and soy sauce in a medium bowl, and toss to coat. Remove from the oven and push the chicken to the sides of the dish. Brush the remaining sweet-and-sour sauce over the chicken and arrange the vegetable mixture in the center of the dish. Bake for 12 to 15 minutes more, stirring vegetables halfway through the cooking process. On each serving plate, arrange 1 thigh and 1 cup vegetables over ½ cup brown rice. Serves 4.

Nutritional Information: 388 calories; 5g fat (12% calories from fat); 32g protein; 53g carbohydrate; 5g dietary fiber; 66mg cholesterol; 418mg sodium.

DAY 6

Breakfast

Raspberry-banana Smoothie

1 6-oz. container artificially sweetened vanilla-flavored nonfat yogurt
½ small banana

¼ cup raspberries
½ cup orange juice

Combine all ingredients in blender and blend well. Serve with 1 slice whole-wheat toast topped with 1 slice 2%-milk sharp cheddar cheese. Serves 1.

Nutritional Information: 212 calories; 1g fat (3.9% calories from fat); 9g protein; 44g carbohydrate; 5g dietary fiber; 2mg cholesterol; 100mg sodium.

Lunch

1 Arby's Light Roast Chicken Deluxe Sandwich®

1 side garden salad with 2 tbsp. lowfat salad dressing and 1 small apple

Nutritional Information: 649 calories; 31g fat (42.2% calories from fat); 28g protein; 68g carbohydrate; 9g dietary fiber; 47mg cholesterol; 1,252mg sodium.

Dinner

Bowtie Pasta with Ham and Asparagus

8 oz. cooked lean ham slices, cut into thin strips

2 cups bowtie pasta
1 10-oz. pkg. frozen cut asparagus

1 8-oz. container light cream cheese
  with chives and onion

$^1/_3$ cup nonfat milk
4 tsp. freshly grated Parmesan cheese

Cook pasta according to package directions, omitting salt and oil. During the last 5 minutes of the cooking time, add asparagus to the pasta. Drain and return to pan. In a small bowl, combine cream cheese and milk. Blend well and set aside. Toss the ham with the pasta mixture and gently stir in cream-cheese mixture over medium heat until thoroughly heated. Divide evenly among 4 bowls and sprinkle each with 1 teaspoon Parmesan cheese. Serve each with 2 servings *Green Beans Italiano* and a 2" slice of French bread. Serves 4.

Nutritional Information: 432 calories; 14g fat (30% calories from fat); 27g protein; 48g carbohydrate; 3g dietary fiber; 60mg cholesterol; 1,180mg sodium.

Green Beans Italiano
1 12-oz. pkg. frozen Italian-cut green beans
1 cup prepared marinara sauce

In a medium saucepan, prepare green beans according to package direction. Drain the green beans and return to the pan. Add marinara and heat through over medium heat. Serves 4.

Nutritional Information: 64 calories; 1g fat (19.1% calories from fat); 2g protein; 12g carbohydrate; 3g dietary fiber; 0mg cholesterol; 260mg sodium.

DAY 7

....

Breakfast
2 lowfat Eggo® frozen waffles
1 cup nonfat milk

½ cup unsweetened applesauce,
  mixed with 1 packet Splenda®
  sugar substitute and
  ½ cup raspberries

Nutritional Information: 345 calories; 6g fat (16.2% calories from fat); 13g protein; 60g carbohydrate; 7g dietary fiber; 27mg cholesterol; 652mg sodium.

....

Lunch
Ranch-style Chicken Fingers
¾ lb. skinless, boneless chicken
  breasts, cut into thin strips

1¾ cup cornflakes crumbs
1 tsp. dried basil

½ cup lowfat buttermilk Ranch salad
  dressing

nonstick cooking spray

Lightly coat a 15″ x 10″ baking pan with nonstick cooking spray and set aside. Preheat oven to 425° F. Combine cornflakes crumbs and basil in shallow dish, and then mix well and set aside. Place the chicken strips in a medium bowl. Add salad dressing and stir to coat. Remove the chicken strips one at a time and roll in the crumb mixture. Arrange the coated strips on a prepared baking pan. Once all of the strips are arranged on the pan, coat lightly with nonstick cooking spray. Bake for 12 to 15 minutes or until the chicken is cooked through. Serve with ½ cup prepared marinara and 2 cups salad made of dark greens and lowfat dressing. Serves 4.

Nutritional Information: 367 calories; 7g fat (17% calories from fat); 27g protein; 51g carbohydrate; 7g dietary fiber; 51mg cholesterol; 1,244mg sodium.

....

Dinner

Salmon with Basil Hollandaise

4 5-oz. skinless center-cut salmon
  fillets
½ cup prepared hollandaise sauce
1 slice day-old bread, toasted and
  crumbled

2 tbsp. basil pesto
1 tbsp. freshly grated Parmesan
  cheese
nonstick cooking spray

Preheat oven to 425° F. Arrange fish on a baking sheet coated with nonstick cooking spray. Bake for 10 to 12 minutes, or until fish flakes easily. Combine bread crumbs, hollandaise, pesto and Parmesan cheese in a small bowl. Stir well and divide mixture evenly over the fillets. Return the fish to the oven and bake for 1 to 2 minutes more. Serve with 1 serving each *Roasted Potatoes* and *Dilly Carrots*. Serves 4.

Nutritional Information: 256 calories; 12g fat (41.6% calories from fat); 31g protein; 5g carbohydrate; trace dietary fiber; 86mg cholesterol; 408mg sodium.

Roasted Potatoes

1½ lbs. red potatoes, each cut into
  wedges
2 tsp. olive oil

½ tsp. rosemary, crumbled
$1/_8$ tsp. pepper
nonstick cooking spray

Preheat oven to 450° F. In a medium bowl, combine potatoes, olive oil, rosemary and pepper, and toss to coat. Spoon mixture into 2-quart baking dish that has been coated with nonstick cooking spray. Bake for 40 minutes or until tender, stirring occasionally. Serves 4 (serving size is 12 wedges).

Nutritional Information: 155 calories; 2g fat (13.8% calories from fat); 4g protein; 31g carbohydrate; 3g dietary fiber; 0mg cholesterol; 10mg sodium.

Dilly Carrots

1 lb. baby carrots
½ tsp. salt

1 tsp. light margarine
1 tsp. dried dill

Place carrots and salt in a medium saucepan and cover with water. Bring the carrots to a boil and cook for 5 minutes or until tender. Drain the carrots and return to pan, and then stir in margarine and dill. Serves 4.

Nutritional Information: 48 calories; 1g fat (11.4% calories from fat); 1g protein; 10g carbohydrate; 3g dietary fiber; 0mg cholesterol; 314mg sodium.

Second Week Grocery List

Produce
- [ ] apples
- [ ] bananas
- [ ] bay leaf
- [ ] broccoli
- [ ] cabbage with carrots, shredded (1 pkg.)
- [ ] capers
- [ ] celery
- [ ] corn
- [ ] grape tomatoes
- [ ] green bell pepper
- [ ] green grapes
- [ ] green onions
- [ ] lemons
- [ ] mushrooms
- [ ] onion
- [ ] onion, sweet
- [ ] red potatoes
- [ ] Romaine lettuce
- [ ] spinach
- [ ] strawberries
- [ ] sugar sweet peas
- [ ] sweet potatoes
- [ ] tomatoes
- [ ] zucchini

Baking/Cooking Products
- [ ] all-fruit spread, apricot
- [ ] apple cider vinegar
- [ ] bacon bits
- [ ] baking powder
- [ ] baking soda
- [ ] balsamic vinaigrette salad dressing, light

- [ ] basil, dried
- [ ] basil pesto
- [ ] butter-flavored flakes
- [ ] buttermilk
- [ ] buttermilk biscuits
- [ ] celery seeds
- [ ] cocktail sauce
- [ ] cornmeal, yellow
- [ ] Dijon mustard
- [ ] dill, dried
- [ ] flour
- [ ] fruit bits, dried
- [ ] ginger, ground
- [ ] honey
- [ ] Italian salad dressing
- [ ] lemon-pepper seasoning
- [ ] liquid crab boil
- [ ] mayonnaise, light
- [ ] nonstick cooking spray
- [ ] olive oil
- [ ] oregano, dried
- [ ] peanut butter
- [ ] pepper, black
- [ ] poppy seed dressing
- [ ] raisins
- [ ] rice, white
- [ ] salad dressing, light
- [ ] salsa
- [ ] salt
- [ ] seafood seasoning
- [ ] sweet-pickle relish
- [ ] vegetable oil
- [ ] yellow rice mix, saffron-flavored

Breads and Cereals
- bread, whole wheat
- cornflakes
- Cream of Wheat,® instant
- dinner rolls, whole grain
- flour tortillas
- grits
- Italian bread
- pasta shells
- pita bread rounds
- Quaker Extra Instant Oatmeal®
- saltine crackers

Canned Foods
- Campbell's Healthy Request Cream of Chicken Soup®
- Campbell's Healthy Request Cream of Mushroom Soup®
- Chicken of the Sea® skinless, boneless pink salmon
- chunk tuna packed in water
- Dole® tropical fruit in juice
- green chilies, undrained
- Healthy Choice Garden Vegetable Soup®
- olives
- petite-diced tomatoes
- refried beans

Dairy Products
- cheddar cheese, sharp 2%
- margarine, light
- Mediterranean-style feta cheese
- milk, nonfat
- Parmesan cheese
- sour cream

Juices
- orange juice

Frozen Foods
- corn, whole-kernel
- creamed spinach
- hash brown potatoes, southwestern-style
- Healthy Choice Chicken Teriyaki Entrée®
- Hormel® beef tips with gravy
- Lean Cuisine Cheese Lasagna with Chicken Scaloppini Entrée®
- Lean Cuisine Deluxe French Bread Pizza®
- mixed vegetables
- sugar snap peas

Meat and Poultry
- deli-roasted chicken
- eggs
- egg substitute
- shrimp
- tilapia
- turkey breast cutlets
- turkey sausage

Second Week Meals and Recipes

DAY 1

Breakfast

1 cup prepared grits, mixed with
  1 slice 2% sharp cheddar cheese

½ cup nonfat milk
1 small banana

Nutritional Information: 477 calories; 9g fat (17% calories from fat); 35g protein; 65g carbohydrate; 3g dietary fiber; 25mg cholesterol; 735mg sodium.

Lunch

11-oz. Healthy Choice Chicken
  Teriyaki Entrée®

1 cup sliced strawberries, tossed with
  1 tbsp. prepared poppy seed dressing

Nutritional Information: 330 calories; 5g fat (12.6% calories from fat); 16g protein; 56g carbohydrate; 12g dietary fiber; 25mg cholesterol; 552mg sodium.

Dinner

Fish Fillets Florentine au Gratin

4 5-oz. tilapia fillets
¼ tsp. lemon-pepper seasoning
1 10-oz. frozen creamed spinach,
  thawed

¼ cup fine dry Italian bread crumbs
¼ cup shredded 2% cheddar cheese
nonstick cooking spray

Preheat oven to 400° F. Season fillets with lemon-pepper seasoning, arrange on a baking sheet coated with nonstick cooking spray, and set aside. In a small bowl, combine thawed spinach with bread crumbs. Spoon mixture evenly over the fillets and bake for 15 minutes or until fish flakes easily. Top each fillet with 1 tablespoon cheese and bake for 1 to 2 minutes more or until cheese is melted. Serve each with 1 serving *Sweet Potatoes and Sugar Snap Peas* and 1 whole-grain dinner roll. Serves 4.

Nutritional Information: 283 calories; 12g fat (42.3% calories from fat); 28g protein; 10g carbohydrate; 1g dietary fiber; 82mg cholesterol; 590mg sodium.

Sweet Potatoes and Sugar Snap Peas

2 large sweet potatoes (about 1 lb.
  each), peeled and cubed

1 10-oz. pkg. frozen sugar snap peas,
  thawed

½ tsp. salt, divided   ½ tsp. dried dill
2 tsp. olive oil

Cover potatoes with water in medium saucepan and add ¼ teaspoon salt.
Bring to boil and simmer for 10 to 12 minutes or until potatoes are tender.
Drain and set aside, keeping warm. In medium skillet, sauté snap peas in
olive oil for 3 minutes, and then stir in dill and remaining salt. Toss peas
with potatoes. Serves 4.

Nutritional Information: 143 calories; 3g fat (16.7% calories from fat); 5g protein; 26g carbohydrate; 5g dietary fiber; 0mg cholesterol; 355mg sodium.

DAY 2

Breakfast
1½ cups cornflakes   1 cup sliced strawberries
1 cup nonfat milk

Nutritional Information: 289 calories; 1g fat (4% calories from fat); 12g protein; 60g carbohydrate; 5g dietary fiber; 4mg cholesterol; 575mg sodium.

Lunch

Tex-Mex Salmon-Potato Cakes

2 7.1-oz. pouches Chicken of the Sea®   ½ cup egg substitute
  skinless, boneless pink salmon   2 tsp. seafood seasoning
2 cups refrigerated southwestern-   4 tsp. olive oil, divided
  style shredded hash brown   ½ cup cocktail sauce
  potatoes   nonstick cooking spray

Remove fish from the pouch, rinse and pat dry with paper towel. Place in a
large skillet and then add just enough water to cover the top of the fish.
Bring to a boil, and then reduce heat to simmer and cook for 8 to 10 minutes or until fish begins to flake easily. Remove fish from the skillet and
allow to cool slightly. Flake the fish into medium bowl. Add hash brown
potatoes, egg substitute and seafood seasoning, and then stir gently to combine. Shape mixture into 8 patties and refrigerate for 15 to 20 minutes.
When the patties are chilled, coat both sides with nonstick cooking spray
and set aside. Preheat a large nonstick skillet over medium-high heat and

add 2 teaspoons olive oil. Place 4 patties into the skillet and cook over medium-high heat for 2 to 3 minutes on each side or until browned and heated through. Remove cakes from the skillet and keep warm. Add the remaining olive oil to the skillet and cook the remaining patties in the same manner. Serve immediately or refrigerate for later use. Serve with 1 tablespoon cocktail sauce and 1 cup steamed broccoli florets. Serves 4.

Nutritional Information: 327 calories; 15g fat (40.4% calories from fat); 26g protein; 23g carbohydrate; 2g dietary fiber; 56mg cholesterol; 762mg sodium.

Dinner

½ order chicken or steak fajitas from your favorite restaurant
2 flour tortillas

½ cup refried beans
½ cup salsa
1 tsp. sour cream

Nutritional Information: 387 calories; 12g fat (34.1% calories from fat); 6g protein; 45g carbohydrate; 5g dietary fiber; 1mg cholesterol; 1,322mg sodium.

DAY 3

Breakfast

1 packet instant Cream of Wheat®
1 slice whole-wheat toast

1 tsp. light margarine
1 cup nonfat milk

Nutritional Information: 388 calories; 4g fat (10% calories from fat); 17g protein; 70g carbohydrate; 4g dietary fiber; 4mg cholesterol; 329mg sodium.

Lunch

1 cup Healthy Choice Garden Vegetable Soup®
1 small banana

peanut-butter sandwich, made with 2 slices whole-wheat bread and 1 tbsp. peanut butter

Nutritional Information: 462 calories; 12g fat (21.4% calories from fat); 16g protein; 81g carbohydrate; 13g dietary fiber; 5mg cholesterol; 852mg sodium.

Dinner

Old-Fashioned Shrimp Boil

1½ lbs. shrimp with shells on, heads off

2 lemons, quartered
2 tbsp. liquid crab boil

2 tbsp. olive oil
1 bay leaf
1 large onion, quartered
2 tbsp. salt

8 small red potatoes, halved
4 small (4″) ears of corn
ice

Squeeze the lemons into large cooking pot. Toss the rinds into a pan and add the liquid crab boil, olive oil, bay leaf, onion, salt, potatoes and corn. Add enough water to cover the mixture, and then add 4 more cups of water. Bring to a boil, and continue boiling for 5 minutes. Add shrimp and continue boiling for 2 minutes more. Add enough ice to the pot to stop the cooking process. Allow to sit for 15 minutes, and then strain and keep warm. Serve each with ¼ cup cocktail sauce and 1 serving *Easy Coleslaw*. Serves 4. (Serving size is 9 to 10 shrimp, 4 potato halves and 1 ear of corn.)

Nutritional Information: 393 calories; 11g fat (24.1% calories from fat); 39g protein; 37g carbohydrate; 4g dietary fiber; 259mg cholesterol; 3,469mg sodium.

Easy Coleslaw
1 16-oz. pkg. shredded cabbage with
  carrots
1 cup light mayonnaise
¼ cup apple cider vinegar

1 tbsp. honey
1 tsp. celery seeds
¼ cup raisins

Place cabbage mixture into a large bowl and set aside. In a small bowl, combine mayonnaise, vinegar and honey. Blend well and pour over the cabbage. Toss to coat, add celery seeds and raisins, and then toss again. Refrigerate until ready to serve. Serves 8.

Nutritional Information: 107 calories; 6g fat (46.8% calories from fat); 1g protein; 14g carbohydrate; 2g dietary fiber; 11mg cholesterol; 160mg sodium.

DAY 4

Breakfast
1 packet Quaker Extra Instant
  Oatmeal®
1 slice whole-wheat toast

½ medium banana
1 tsp. peanut butter
1 cup nonfat milk

Nutritional Information: 358 calories; 4g fat (10.6% calories from fat); 18g protein; 65g carbohydrate; 8g dietary fiber; 4mg cholesterol; 683mg sodium.

Lunch

Quick and Easy Beef Stew

1 17-oz. pkg. refrigerated Hormel®
  beef tips with gravy
2 10.75-oz. cans Campbell's Healthy
  Request Cream of Mushroom Soup®

1 14.5-oz. can petite-diced tomatoes
1 16-oz. pkg. frozen mixed vegetables
1 cup nonfat milk
1 tsp. dried basil

Bring beef tips with gravy, mushroom soup, tomatoes (with liquid), vegetables, milk and basil to a boil in large saucepan, stirring occasionally. Serve hot. Serve with 1 serving *Kickin' Skillet Cornbread*. Serves 4.

Nutritional Information: 405 calories; 16g fat (35.1% calories from fat); 12g protein; 55g carbohydrate; 8g dietary fiber; 4mg cholesterol; 1,826mg sodium.

Kickin' Skillet Cornbread

3 tsp. vegetable oil, divided
1 cup yellow cornmeal
¾ cup flour
1½ tsp. baking powder
¼ tsp. baking soda
¼ tsp. salt

¾ cup buttermilk
1 4-oz. can chopped green chilies,
  undrained
¼ cup egg substitute
½ cup frozen whole kernel corn,
  thawed

Preheat oven to 400° F. Coat an 8″ cast-iron skillet with 1 teaspoon oil and place in the oven for 10 minutes. Combine cornmeal, flour, baking powder, baking soda and salt in a large bowl. Mix well and set aside. In a small bowl, combine the remaining oil, buttermilk, chilies and egg substitute. Mix well and then add to the cornmeal mixture, stirring until the dry ingredients are moistened. Stir in corn and mix well. Spoon the mixture onto a preheated skillet and bake for 45 minutes or until a wooden pick inserted in the center of the cornbread comes out clean. Serves 10.

Nutritional Information: 125 calories; 3g fat (18.6% calories from fat); 4g protein; 22g carbohydrate; 2g dietary fiber; 1mg cholesterol; 191mg sodium.

Dinner

10-oz. Lean Cuisine Cheese Lasagna
  with Chicken Scaloppini Entrée®
1 cup spinach salad, with
sliced tomatoes

sliced mushrooms
1 tsp. bacon bits
2 tbsp. light salad dressing
4 saltine crackers

Nutritional Information: 456 calories; 14g fat (27.4% calories from fat); 19g protein; 64g carbohydrate; 6g dietary fiber; 22mg cholesterol; 1,252mg sodium.

DAY 5

....

Breakfast

Biscuits with Sausage Gravy

6 oz. bulk turkey sausage
1 7.5-oz. can (10 ct.) reduced-fat
   buttermilk biscuits
2 cups nonfat milk

2 tbsp. flour
2 tsp. butter-flavored flakes
¼ tsp. black pepper
nonstick cooking spray

Preheat oven to 450° F. Arrange biscuits on a nonstick baking sheet and set aside. Heat a skillet coated with nonstick cooking spray over medium heat. Crumble sausage into the skillet and cook until thoroughly done. Drain any visible fat, and then return the sausage to the skillet. When the sausage is nearly done, combine milk, flour, butter-flavored flakes and pepper in medium bowl. Mix well and add to the skillet with the sausage. Cook for 8 minutes or until thickened, stirring occasionally with a spatula to prevent sticking. As the gravy is cooking, place biscuits in the oven, and bake for 5 to 6 minutes or until done. Split biscuits and arrange 4 halves on each serving plate. Top each biscuit with ½ cup sausage gravy. Serve with ¾ cup orange juice. Serves 5.

Nutritional Information: 386 calories; 16g fat (37.7% calories from fat); 12g protein; 48g carbohydrate; 1g dietary fiber; 25mg cholesterol; 810mg sodium.

....

Lunch

1 Lean Cuisine Deluxe French Bread Pizza®
1 serving *Easy Coleslaw* (see Day 3 dinner recipe)

Nutritional Information: 554 calories; 22g fat (34.8% calories from fat); 18g protein; 74g carbohydrate; 7g dietary fiber; 42mg cholesterol; 1,081mg sodium.

....

Dinner

Turkey Piccata

1 lb. turkey breast cutlets
½ cup light Italian salad dressing,
   divided
2 tbsp. light mayonnaise

2 tsp. finely shredded lemon peel
juice from 1 lemon
dash of black pepper
1 tbsp. capers, rinsed

Place cutlets and ¼ cup salad dressing into sealable plastic bag. Seal and re-frigerate for 2 to 3 hours or overnight. When ready to use, preheat oven to 425° F and arrange cutlets on a nonstick baking sheet. Bake the cutlets for 12 to 15 minutes, and then remove from the oven. In small bowl, combine the remaining salad dressing, mayonnaise, lemon peel, lemon juice, black pepper and capers, and then top each cutlet with 1 tablespoon of the sauce. Serve each with 1 serving *Baked Veggie Risotto*. Serves 4.

Nutritional Information: 185 calories; 7g fat (35.4% calories from fat); 24g protein; 5g carbo-hydrate; trace dietary fiber; 75mg cholesterol; 396mg sodium.

Baked Veggie Risotto

1 10.75-oz. can condensed Campbell's Healthy Request Cream of Chicken Soup®	½ cup diced sweet onion
	1 10-oz. pkg. frozen sugar snap peas
1 cup white rice	¼ tsp. coarsely ground black pepper
½ cup shredded carrots	2 tbsp. freshly grated Parmesan cheese

Preheat oven to 375° F. Place 3 cups water, soup, rice, carrots and onion into a 2-quart casserole dish. Stir to combine the ingredients. Bake, covered, for 55 minutes, and then remove from the oven and stir in sugar snap peas and pepper. Cook for 5 minutes more. Remove from the oven and gently stir in cheese. Let stand for 5 minutes before serving. Serves 4.

Nutritional Information: 320 calories; 6g fat (16.5% calories from fat); 11g protein; 56g car-bohydrate; 5g dietary fiber; 8mg cholesterol; 738mg sodium.

DAY 6

Breakfast

1 egg, poached or cooked with butter-flavored nonstick cooking spray	1 small apple
	1 cup nonfat milk
2 slices whole-wheat toast	

Nutritional Information: 370 calories; 8g fat (18% calories from fat); 20g protein; 59g carbo-hydrate; 8g dietary fiber; 191mg cholesterol; 477mg sodium.

Lunch

Mediterranean-Style Seafood and Pasta Salad

6 oz. cooked salad shrimp	1 cup halved grape tomatoes
1½ cups miniature pasta shells	1 cup diced zucchini

½ cup sliced mushrooms
¼ cup ripe olives
4 oz. Mediterranean-style feta cheese, crumbled

½ cup light balsamic vinaigrette salad dressing
4 cups fresh spinach leaves

Cook pasta according to package directions, omitting salt and fat. Drain and rinse, and then place in a large bowl. Add shrimp, tomatoes, zucchini, mushrooms, olives and feta cheese, and then stir to combine. Add the salad dressing and toss to coat. Arrange 1 cup spinach leaves on each serving plate and top with the shrimp mixture. Serve each with 1 cup green grapes. Serves 4.

Nutritional Information: 364 calories; 8g fat (19.9% calories from fat); 20g protein; 55g carbohydrate; 4g dietary fiber; 108mg cholesterol; 520mg sodium.

Dinner

1 Outback Steakhouse® chicken and veggie or shrimp and veggie griller meal

1 side salad
2 tbsp. light salad dressing

Nutritional Information: 648 calories; 29g fat (61% calories from fat); 3g protein; 39g carbohydrate; 4g dietary fiber; 192mg cholesterol; 1,621mg sodium.

DAY 7

Breakfast

McDonald's Egg McMuffin®   ½ small banana

Nutritional Information: 345 calories; 6g fat (16.2% calories from fat); 13g protein; 60g carbohydrate; 7g dietary fiber; 27mg cholesterol; 652mg sodium.

Lunch

Tuna-Veggie Pita Pockets

2 6-in. pita bread rounds, cut in half
1 6^1/$_8$-oz. can chunk tuna packed in water, drained
¼ cup light mayonnaise
^{1}/$_8$ tsp. black pepper

2 tbsp. sweet-pickle relish, drained
2 tsp. Dijon mustard
½ cup coarsely shredded carrots
½ cup finely chopped green bell pepper
^{1}/$_3$ cup finely chopped celery

$^1/_3$ cup thinly sliced green onions,
   tops only

2 cups chopped romaine lettuce
4 thick tomato slices

Combine tuna, mayonnaise, black pepper, relish and mustard in large bowl and stir well. Add carrots, bell pepper, celery and green onions, and toss gently. Spoon equal amounts of the mixture into each pita half. Top each with equal amounts of lettuce and 1 slice tomato. Serve each with ½ cup canned Dole tropical fruit in juice. Serves 4.

Nutritional Information: 338 calories; 5g fat (14% calories from fat); 5g protein; 61g carbohydrate; 6g dietary fiber; 24mg cholesterol; 459mg sodium.

....

Dinner

Roasted Chicken with Fruit and Pesto

1 3½ to 4½ lb. deli roasted chicken
1 cup apricot all-fruit spread
½ cup dried fruit bits

¼ tsp. ground ginger
½ cup basil pesto

Preheat oven to 350° F. Remove skin from the chicken and discard. Strip meat from the bones, place into a 4-quart baking dish, and set aside. In medium bowl, combine fruit spread, fruit bits, ginger and pesto. Stir well and pour over the chicken. Bake for 12 to 15 minutes. Serve each with *Roasted Zucchini*, 1 serving *Fruited Saffron Rice* and 1 wedge *Kickin' Skillet Cornbread* (see the day four lunch recipe for this week). Serves 6.

Nutritional Information: 346 calories; 14g fat (35.7% calories from fat); 21g protein; 34g carbohydrate; 1g dietary fiber; 60mg cholesterol; 193mg sodium.

Roasted Zucchini

3 lbs. small zucchini
2 tsp. olive oil
½ tsp. dried oregano

½ tsp. salt
¼ tsp. black pepper

Preheat oven to 450° F. Slice zucchini in half lengthwise, and then quarter each half. Toss zucchini pieces with oil, oregano, salt and pepper in a large bowl. Arrange in a 4-quart baking dish and bake for 20 to 25 minutes or until tender. Serves 6.

Nutritional Information: 44 calories; 2g fat (31.4% calories from fat); 3g protein; 6g carbohydrate; 3g dietary fiber; 0mg cholesterol; 184mg sodium.

Fruited Saffron Rice
1 5-oz. pkg. saffron-flavored yellow rice mix
½ cup dried fruit bits

Prepare rice according to package directions, adding fruit bits at the beginning. Serves 6.

Nutritional Information: 101 calories; trace fat (4% calories from fat); 3g protein; 22g carbohydrate; 2g dietary fiber; 0mg cholesterol; 403mg sodium.

Member Survey

Please answer the following questions to help your leader plan your First Place 4 Health meetings so that your needs might be met in this session. Give this form to your leader at the first group meeting.

Name _____ Birth date _____

Please list those who live in your household.

Name	Relationship	Age
_____	_____	_____
_____	_____	_____
_____	_____	_____
_____	_____	_____

What church do you attend? _____

Are you interested in receiving more information about our church?

     Yes   No

Occupation _____

What talent or area of expertise would you be willing to share with our class?

_____

Why did you join First Place 4 Health?

_____

With notice, would you be willing to lead a Bible study discussion one week?

     Yes   No

Are you comfortable praying out loud? _____

If the assistant leader were absent, would you be willing to assist in weighing in members and possibly evaluating the Live It Trackers?

     Yes   No

Any other comments:

_____

_____

Personal Weight and Measurement Record

Week	Weight	+ or -	Goal this Session	Pounds to goal
1				
2				
3				
4				
5				
6				
7				
8				
9				
10				
11				
12				

Beginning Measurements

Waist _____ Hips _____ Thighs _____ Chest _____

Ending Measurements

Waist _____ Hips _____ Thighs _____ Chest _____

First Place 4 Health
Prayer Partner

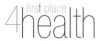

WALKING IN
GRACE
Week
5

This righteousness from God comes through faith in Jesus Christ to all who believe. There is no difference, for all have sinned and fall short of the glory of God, and are justified freely by his grace through the redemption that came by Christ Jesus.

ROMANS 3:22-24

Date: _____

Name: _____

Home Phone: (_____) _____

Work Phone: (_____) _____

Email: _____

Personal Prayer Concerns:

_____

_____

_____

_____

_____

_____

_____

This form is for prayer requests that are personal to you and your journey in First Place 4 Health. Please complete this form and have it ready to turn in when you arrive at your group meeting.

First Place 4 Health
Prayer Partner

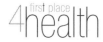

WALKING IN
GRACE
Week
7

<small>SCRIPTURE VERSE TO MEMORIZE FOR WEEK EIGHT:</small>

The name of the Lord is a strong tower; the righteous run to it and are safe.

<small>PROVERBS 18:10</small>

Date: _____

Name: _____

Home Phone: (_____) _____

Work Phone: (_____) _____

Email: _____

Personal Prayer Concerns:

_____

_____

_____

_____

_____

_____

_____

This form is for prayer requests that are personal to you and your journey in First Place 4 Health. Please complete this form and have it ready to turn in when you arrive at your group meeting.

First Place 4 Health
Prayer Partner

WALKING IN
GRACE
Week
9

Scripture Verse to Memorize for Week Ten:

And whatever you do, whether in word or deed, do it all in the name of the Lord Jesus, giving thanks to God the Father through Him.

Colossians 3:17

Date:

Name:

Home Phone: (   )

Work Phone: (   )

Email:

Personal Prayer Concerns:

_____

_____

_____

_____

_____

_____

_____

_____

This form is for prayer requests that are personal to you and your journey in First Place 4 Health. Please complete this form and have it ready to turn in when you arrive at your group meeting.

Live It Tracker

Name: _____ Loss/gain: _____ lbs.

Date: _____ Week #: _____ Calorie Range: _____ My food goal for next week: _____

Activity Level: None, < 30 min/day, 30-60 min/day, 60+ min/day My activity goal for next week: _____

Group	Daily Calories							
	1300-1400	1500-1600	1700-1800	1900-2000	2100-2200	2300-2400	2500-2600	2700-2800
Fruits	1.5-2 c.	1.5-2 c.	1.5-2 c.	2-2.5 c.	2-2.5 c.	2.5-3.5 c.	3.5-4.5 c.	3.5-4.5 c.
Vegetables	1.5-2 c.	2-2.5 c.	2.5-3 c.	2.5-3 c.	3-3.5 c.	3.5-4.5 c.	4.5-5 c.	4.5-5 c.
Grains	5 oz-eq.	5-6 oz-eq.	6-7 oz-eq.	6-7 oz-eq.	7-8 oz-eq.	8-9 oz-eq.	9-10 oz-eq.	10-11 oz-eq.
Meat & Beans	4 oz-eq.	5 oz-eq.	5-5.5 oz-eq.	5.5-6.5 oz-eq.	6.5-7 oz-eq.	7-7.5 oz-eq.	7-7.5 oz-eq.	7.5-8 oz-eq.
Milk	2-3 c.	3 c.	3 c.	3 c.	3 c.	3 c.	3 c.	3 c.
Healthy Oils	4 tsp.	5 tsp.	5 tsp.	6 tsp.	6 tsp.	7 tsp.	8 tsp.	8 tsp.

Day/Date:

Breakfast: _____ Lunch: _____

Dinner: _____ Snack: _____

Group	Fruits	Vegetables	Grains	Meat & Beans	Milk	Oils
Goal Amount						
Estimate Your Total						
Increase ⇧ or Decrease? ⇩						

Physical Activity: _____ Spiritual Activity: _____

Steps/Miles/Minutes: _____

Day/Date:

Breakfast: _____ Lunch: _____

Dinner: _____ Snack: _____

Group	Fruits	Vegetables	Grains	Meat & Beans	Milk	Oils
Goal Amount						
Estimate Your Total						
Increase ⇧ or Decrease? ⇩						

Physical Activity: _____ Spiritual Activity: _____

Steps/Miles/Minutes: _____

Day/Date:

Breakfast: _____ Lunch: _____

Dinner: _____ Snack: _____

Group	Fruits	Vegetables	Grains	Meat & Beans	Milk	Oils
Goal Amount						
Estimate Your Total						
Increase ⇧ or Decrease? ⇩						

Physical Activity: _____ Spiritual Activity: _____

Steps/Miles/Minutes: _____

Day/Date: ____

Breakfast: _____   Lunch: _____

Dinner: _____   Snack: _____

Group	Fruits	Vegetables	Grains	Meat & Beans	Milk	Oils
Goal Amount						
Estimate Your Total						
Increase ⇧ or Decrease? ⇩						

Physical Activity: _____   Spiritual Activity: _____

Steps/Miles/Minutes: _____   _____

Day/Date: ____

Breakfast: _____   Lunch: _____

Dinner: _____   Snack: _____

Group	Fruits	Vegetables	Grains	Meat & Beans	Milk	Oils
Goal Amount						
Estimate Your Total						
Increase ⇧ or Decrease? ⇩						

Physical Activity: _____   Spiritual Activity: _____

Steps/Miles/Minutes: _____   _____

Day/Date: ____

Breakfast: _____   Lunch: _____

Dinner: _____   Snack: _____

Group	Fruits	Vegetables	Grains	Meat & Beans	Milk	Oils
Goal Amount						
Estimate Your Total						
Increase ⇧ or Decrease? ⇩						

Physical Activity: _____   Spiritual Activity: _____

Steps/Miles/Minutes: _____   _____

Day/Date: ____

Breakfast: _____   Lunch: _____

Dinner: _____   Snack: _____

Group	Fruits	Vegetables	Grains	Meat & Beans	Milk	Oils
Goal Amount						
Estimate Your Total						
Increase ⇧ or Decrease? ⇩						

Physical Activity: _____   Spiritual Activity: _____

Steps/Miles/Minutes: _____   _____

Live It Tracker

Name: _____ Loss/gain: _____ lbs.

Date: _____ Week #: ____ Calorie Range: _____ My food goal for next week: _____

Activity Level: None, < 30 min/day, 30-60 min/day, 60+ min/day My activity goal for next week: _____

Group	Daily Calories							
	1300-1400	1500-1600	1700-1800	1900-2000	2100-2200	2300-2400	2500-2600	2700-2800
Fruits	1.5-2 c.	1.5-2 c.	1.5-2 c.	2-2.5 c.	2-2.5 c.	2.5-3.5 c.	3.5-4.5 c.	3.5-4.5 c.
Vegetables	1.5-2 c.	2-2.5 c.	2.5-3 c.	2.5-3 c.	3-3.5 c.	3.5-4.5 c.	4.5-5 c.	4.5-5 c.
Grains	5 oz-eq.	5-6 oz-eq.	6-7 oz-eq.	6-7 oz-eq.	7-8 oz-eq.	8-9 oz-eq.	9-10 oz-eq.	10-11 oz-eq.
Meat & Beans	4 oz-eq.	5 oz-eq.	5-5.5 oz-eq.	5.5-6.5 oz-eq.	6.5-7 oz-eq.	7-7.5 oz-eq.	7-7.5 oz-eq.	7.5-8 oz-eq.
Milk	2-3 c.	3 c.	3 c.	3 c.	3 c.	3 c.	3 c.	3 c.
Healthy Oils	4 tsp.	5 tsp.	5 tsp.	6 tsp.	6 tsp.	7 tsp.	8 tsp.	8 tsp.

Day/Date: ___

Breakfast: _____ Lunch: _____

Dinner: _____ Snack: _____

Group	Fruits	Vegetables	Grains	Meat & Beans	Milk	Oils
Goal Amount						
Estimate Your Total						
Increase ⇧ or Decrease? ⇩						

Physical Activity: _____ Spiritual Activity: _____

Steps/Miles/Minutes: _____

Day/Date: ___

Breakfast: _____ Lunch: _____

Dinner: _____ Snack: _____

Group	Fruits	Vegetables	Grains	Meat & Beans	Milk	Oils
Goal Amount						
Estimate Your Total						
Increase ⇧ or Decrease? ⇩						

Physical Activity: _____ Spiritual Activity: _____

Steps/Miles/Minutes: _____

Day/Date: ___

Breakfast: _____ Lunch: _____

Dinner: _____ Snack: _____

Group	Fruits	Vegetables	Grains	Meat & Beans	Milk	Oils
Goal Amount						
Estimate Your Total						
Increase ⇧ or Decrease? ⇩						

Physical Activity: _____ Spiritual Activity: _____

Steps/Miles/Minutes: _____

Day/Date: _____

Breakfast: _____ Lunch: _____

Dinner: _____ Snack: _____

Group	Fruits	Vegetables	Grains	Meat & Beans	Milk	Oils
Goal Amount						
Estimate Your Total						
Increase ⇧ or Decrease? ⇩						

Physical Activity: _____ Spiritual Activity: _____

Steps/Miles/Minutes: _____

Day/Date: _____

Breakfast: _____ Lunch: _____

Dinner: _____ Snack: _____

Group	Fruits	Vegetables	Grains	Meat & Beans	Milk	Oils
Goal Amount						
Estimate Your Total						
Increase ⇧ or Decrease? ⇩						

Physical Activity: _____ Spiritual Activity: _____

Steps/Miles/Minutes: _____

Day/Date: _____

Breakfast: _____ Lunch: _____

Dinner: _____ Snack: _____

Group	Fruits	Vegetables	Grains	Meat & Beans	Milk	Oils
Goal Amount						
Estimate Your Total						
Increase ⇧ or Decrease? ⇩						

Physical Activity: _____ Spiritual Activity: _____

Steps/Miles/Minutes: _____

Day/Date: _____

Breakfast: _____ Lunch: _____

Dinner: _____ Snack: _____

Group	Fruits	Vegetables	Grains	Meat & Beans	Milk	Oils
Goal Amount						
Estimate Your Total						
Increase ⇧ or Decrease? ⇩						

Physical Activity: _____ Spiritual Activity: _____

Steps/Miles/Minutes: _____

Live It Tracker

Name: _____ Loss/gain: _____ lbs.

Date: _____ Week #: _____ Calorie Range: _____ My food goal for next week: _____

Activity Level: None, < 30 min/day, 30-60 min/day, 60+ min/day My activity goal for next week: _____

Group	Daily Calories							
	1300-1400	1500-1600	1700-1800	1900-2000	2100-2200	2300-2400	2500-2600	2700-2800
Fruits	1.5-2 c.	1.5-2 c.	1.5-2 c.	2-2.5 c.	2-2.5 c.	2.5-3.5 c.	3.5-4.5 c.	3.5-4.5 c.
Vegetables	1.5-2 c.	2-2.5 c.	2.5-3 c.	2.5-3 c.	3-3.5 c.	3.5-4.5 c.	4.5-5 c.	4.5-5 c.
Grains	5 oz-eq.	5-6 oz-eq.	6-7 oz-eq.	6-7 oz-eq.	7-8 oz-eq.	8-9 oz-eq.	9-10 oz-eq.	10-11 oz-eq.
Meat & Beans	4 oz-eq.	5 oz-eq.	5-5.5 oz-eq.	5.5-6.5 oz-eq.	6.5-7 oz-eq.	7-7.5 oz-eq.	7-7.5 oz-eq.	7.5-8 oz-eq.
Milk	2-3 c.	3 c.	3 c.	3 c.	3 c.	3 c.	3 c.	3 c.
Healthy Oils	4 tsp.	5 tsp.	5 tsp.	6 tsp.	6 tsp.	7 tsp.	8 tsp.	8 tsp.

Day/Date: _____

Breakfast: _____   Lunch: _____

Dinner: _____   Snack: _____

Group	Fruits	Vegetables	Grains	Meat & Beans	Milk	Oils
Goal Amount						
Estimate Your Total						
Increase ⇧ or Decrease? ⇩						

Physical Activity: _____   Spiritual Activity: _____

Steps/Miles/Minutes: _____

Day/Date: _____

Breakfast: _____   Lunch: _____

Dinner: _____   Snack: _____

Group	Fruits	Vegetables	Grains	Meat & Beans	Milk	Oils
Goal Amount						
Estimate Your Total						
Increase ⇧ or Decrease? ⇩						

Physical Activity: _____   Spiritual Activity: _____

Steps/Miles/Minutes: _____

Day/Date: _____

Breakfast: _____   Lunch: _____

Dinner: _____   Snack: _____

Group	Fruits	Vegetables	Grains	Meat & Beans	Milk	Oils
Goal Amount						
Estimate Your Total						
Increase ⇧ or Decrease? ⇩						

Physical Activity: _____   Spiritual Activity: _____

Steps/Miles/Minutes: _____

Day/Date:

Breakfast: _____ Lunch: _____

Dinner: _____ Snack: _____

Group	Fruits	Vegetables	Grains	Meat & Beans	Milk	Oils
Goal Amount						
Estimate Your Total						
Increase ⬆ or Decrease? ⬇						

Physical Activity: _____ Spiritual Activity: _____

Steps/Miles/Minutes: _____ _____

Day/Date:

Breakfast: _____ Lunch: _____

Dinner: _____ Snack: _____

Group	Fruits	Vegetables	Grains	Meat & Beans	Milk	Oils
Goal Amount						
Estimate Your Total						
Increase ⬆ or Decrease? ⬇						

Physical Activity: _____ Spiritual Activity: _____

Steps/Miles/Minutes: _____ _____

Day/Date:

Breakfast: _____ Lunch: _____

Dinner: _____ Snack: _____

Group	Fruits	Vegetables	Grains	Meat & Beans	Milk	Oils
Goal Amount						
Estimate Your Total						
Increase ⬆ or Decrease? ⬇						

Physical Activity: _____ Spiritual Activity: _____

Steps/Miles/Minutes: _____ _____

Day/Date:

Breakfast: _____ Lunch: _____

Dinner: _____ Snack: _____

Group	Fruits	Vegetables	Grains	Meat & Beans	Milk	Oils
Goal Amount						
Estimate Your Total						
Increase ⬆ or Decrease? ⬇						

Physical Activity: _____ Spiritual Activity: _____

Steps/Miles/Minutes: _____ _____

Live It Tracker

Name: _____ Loss/gain: _____ lbs.

Date: _____ Week #: ____ Calorie Range: _____ My food goal for next week: _____

Activity Level: None, < 30 min/day, 30-60 min/day, 60+ min/day My activity goal for next week: _____

Group	Daily Calories							
	1300-1400	1500-1600	1700-1800	1900-2000	2100-2200	2300-2400	2500-2600	2700-2800
Fruits	1.5-2 c.	1.5-2 c.	1.5-2 c.	2-2.5 c.	2-2.5 c.	2.5-3.5 c.	3.5-4.5 c.	3.5-4.5 c.
Vegetables	1.5-2 c.	2-2.5 c.	2.5-3 c.	2.5-3 c.	3-3.5 c.	3.5-4.5 c.	4.5-5 c.	4.5-5 c.
Grains	5 oz-eq.	5-6 oz-eq.	6-7 oz-eq.	6-7 oz-eq.	7-8 oz-eq.	8-9 oz-eq.	9-10 oz-eq.	10-11 oz-eq.
Meat & Beans	4 oz-eq.	5 oz-eq.	5-5.5 oz-eq.	5.5-6.5 oz-eq.	6.5-7 oz-eq.	7-7.5 oz-eq.	7-7.5 oz-eq.	7.5-8 oz-eq.
Milk	2-3 c.	3 c.	3 c.	3 c.	3 c.	3 c.	3 c.	3 c.
Healthy Oils	4 tsp.	5 tsp.	5 tsp.	6 tsp.	6 tsp.	7 tsp.	8 tsp.	8 tsp.

Day/Date: ____

Breakfast: _____ Lunch: _____

Dinner: _____ Snack: _____

Group	Fruits	Vegetables	Grains	Meat & Beans	Milk	Oils
Goal Amount						
Estimate Your Total						
Increase ⇧ or Decrease? ⇩						

Physical Activity: _____ Spiritual Activity: _____

Steps/Miles/Minutes: _____

Day/Date: ____

Breakfast: _____ Lunch: _____

Dinner: _____ Snack: _____

Group	Fruits	Vegetables	Grains	Meat & Beans	Milk	Oils
Goal Amount						
Estimate Your Total						
Increase ⇧ or Decrease? ⇩						

Physical Activity: _____ Spiritual Activity: _____

Steps/Miles/Minutes: _____

Day/Date: ____

Breakfast: _____ Lunch: _____

Dinner: _____ Snack: _____

Group	Fruits	Vegetables	Grains	Meat & Beans	Milk	Oils
Goal Amount						
Estimate Your Total						
Increase ⇧ or Decrease? ⇩						

Physical Activity: _____ Spiritual Activity: _____

Steps/Miles/Minutes: _____

Day/Date:

Breakfast: _____ Lunch: _____

Dinner: _____ Snack: _____

Group	Fruits	Vegetables	Grains	Meat & Beans	Milk	Oils
Goal Amount						
Estimate Your Total						
Increase ⇧ or Decrease? ⇩						

Physical Activity: _____ Spiritual Activity: _____

Steps/Miles/Minutes: _____ _____

Day/Date:

Breakfast: _____ Lunch: _____

Dinner: _____ Snack: _____

Group	Fruits	Vegetables	Grains	Meat & Beans	Milk	Oils
Goal Amount						
Estimate Your Total						
Increase ⇧ or Decrease? ⇩						

Physical Activity: _____ Spiritual Activity: _____

Steps/Miles/Minutes: _____ _____

Day/Date:

Breakfast: _____ Lunch: _____

Dinner: _____ Snack: _____

Group	Fruits	Vegetables	Grains	Meat & Beans	Milk	Oils
Goal Amount						
Estimate Your Total						
Increase ⇧ or Decrease? ⇩						

Physical Activity: _____ Spiritual Activity: _____

Steps/Miles/Minutes: _____ _____

Day/Date:

Breakfast: _____ Lunch: _____

Dinner: _____ Snack: _____

Group	Fruits	Vegetables	Grains	Meat & Beans	Milk	Oils
Goal Amount						
Estimate Your Total						
Increase ⇧ or Decrease? ⇩						

Physical Activity: _____ Spiritual Activity: _____

Steps/Miles/Minutes: _____ _____

Live It Tracker

Name: _____ Loss/gain: _____ lbs.

Date: _____ Week #: _____ Calorie Range: _____ My food goal for next week: _____

Activity Level: None, < 30 min/day, 30-60 min/day, 60+ min/day My activity goal for next week: _____

Group	Daily Calories							
	1300-1400	1500-1600	1700-1800	1900-2000	2100-2200	2300-2400	2500-2600	2700-2800
Fruits	1.5-2 c.	1.5-2 c.	1.5-2 c.	2-2.5 c.	2-2.5 c.	2.5-3.5 c.	3.5-4.5 c.	3.5-4.5 c.
Vegetables	1.5-2 c.	2-2.5 c.	2.5-3 c.	2.5-3 c.	3-3.5 c.	3.5-4.5 c.	4.5-5 c.	4.5-5 c.
Grains	5 oz-eq.	5-6 oz-eq.	6-7 oz-eq.	6-7 oz-eq.	7-8 oz-eq.	8-9 oz-eq.	9-10 oz-eq.	10-11 oz-eq.
Meat & Beans	4 oz-eq.	5 oz-eq.	5-5.5 oz-eq.	5.5-6.5 oz-eq.	6.5-7 oz-eq.	7-7.5 oz-eq.	7-7.5 oz-eq.	7.5-8 oz-eq.
Milk	2-3 c.	3 c.	3 c.	3 c.	3 c.	3 c.	3 c.	3 c.
Healthy Oils	4 tsp.	5 tsp.	5 tsp.	6 tsp.	6 tsp.	7 tsp.	8 tsp.	8 tsp.

Day/Date:

Breakfast: _____ Lunch: _____

Dinner: _____ Snack: _____

Group	Fruits	Vegetables	Grains	Meat & Beans	Milk	Oils
Goal Amount						
Estimate Your Total						
Increase ⇧ or Decrease? ⇩						

Physical Activity: _____ Spiritual Activity: _____

Steps/Miles/Minutes: _____ _____

Day/Date:

Breakfast: _____ Lunch: _____

Dinner: _____ Snack: _____

Group	Fruits	Vegetables	Grains	Meat & Beans	Milk	Oils
Goal Amount						
Estimate Your Total						
Increase ⇧ or Decrease? ⇩						

Physical Activity: _____ Spiritual Activity: _____

Steps/Miles/Minutes: _____ _____

Day/Date:

Breakfast: _____ Lunch: _____

Dinner: _____ Snack: _____

Group	Fruits	Vegetables	Grains	Meat & Beans	Milk	Oils
Goal Amount						
Estimate Your Total						
Increase ⇧ or Decrease? ⇩						

Physical Activity: _____ Spiritual Activity: _____

Steps/Miles/Minutes: _____ _____

Day/Date: ______

Breakfast: ______

Lunch: ______

Dinner: ______

Snack: ______

Group	Fruits	Vegetables	Grains	Meat & Beans	Milk	Oils
Goal Amount						
Estimate Your Total						
Increase ⇧ or Decrease? ⇩						

Physical Activity: ______

Spiritual Activity: ______

Steps/Miles/Minutes: ______

Day/Date: ______

Breakfast: ______

Lunch: ______

Dinner: ______

Snack: ______

Group	Fruits	Vegetables	Grains	Meat & Beans	Milk	Oils
Goal Amount						
Estimate Your Total						
Increase ⇧ or Decrease? ⇩						

Physical Activity: ______

Spiritual Activity: ______

Steps/Miles/Minutes: ______

Day/Date: ______

Breakfast: ______

Lunch: ______

Dinner: ______

Snack: ______

Group	Fruits	Vegetables	Grains	Meat & Beans	Milk	Oils
Goal Amount						
Estimate Your Total						
Increase ⇧ or Decrease? ⇩						

Physical Activity: ______

Spiritual Activity: ______

Steps/Miles/Minutes: ______

Day/Date: ______

Breakfast: ______

Lunch: ______

Dinner: ______

Snack: ______

Group	Fruits	Vegetables	Grains	Meat & Beans	Milk	Oils
Goal Amount						
Estimate Your Total						
Increase ⇧ or Decrease? ⇩						

Physical Activity: ______

Spiritual Activity: ______

Steps/Miles/Minutes: ______

Live It Tracker

Name: ______________________ Loss/gain: ________ lbs.

Date: ________ Week #: ____ Calorie Range: __________ My food goal for next week: __________

Activity Level: None, < 30 min/day, 30-60 min/day, 60+ min/day My activity goal for next week: __________

Group	Daily Calories							
	1300-1400	1500-1600	1700-1800	1900-2000	2100-2200	2300-2400	2500-2600	2700-2800
Fruits	1.5-2 c.	1.5-2 c.	1.5-2 c.	2-2.5 c.	2-2.5 c.	2.5-3.5 c.	3.5-4.5 c.	3.5-4.5 c.
Vegetables	1.5-2 c.	2-2.5 c.	2.5-3 c.	2.5-3 c.	3-3.5 c.	3.5-4.5 c.	4.5-5 c.	4.5-5 c.
Grains	5 oz-eq.	5-6 oz-eq.	6-7 oz-eq.	6-7 oz-eq.	7-8 oz-eq.	8-9 oz-eq.	9-10 oz-eq.	10-11 oz-eq.
Meat & Beans	4 oz-eq.	5 oz-eq.	5-5.5 oz-eq.	5.5-6.5 oz-eq.	6.5-7 oz-eq.	7-7.5 oz-eq.	7-7.5 oz-eq.	7.5-8 oz-eq.
Milk	2-3 c.	3 c.	3 c.	3 c.	3 c.	3 c.	3 c.	3 c.
Healthy Oils	4 tsp.	5 tsp.	5 tsp.	6 tsp.	6 tsp.	7 tsp.	8 tsp.	8 tsp.

Day/Date: ________

Breakfast: ____________________ Lunch: ____________________

Dinner: ____________________ Snack: ____________________

Group	Fruits	Vegetables	Grains	Meat & Beans	Milk	Oils
Goal Amount						
Estimate Your Total						
Increase ⇧ or Decrease? ⇩						

Physical Activity: ____________________ Spiritual Activity: ____________________

Steps/Miles/Minutes: ____________________

Day/Date: ________

Breakfast: ____________________ Lunch: ____________________

Dinner: ____________________ Snack: ____________________

Group	Fruits	Vegetables	Grains	Meat & Beans	Milk	Oils
Goal Amount						
Estimate Your Total						
Increase ⇧ or Decrease? ⇩						

Physical Activity: ____________________ Spiritual Activity: ____________________

Steps/Miles/Minutes: ____________________

Day/Date: ________

Breakfast: ____________________ Lunch: ____________________

Dinner: ____________________ Snack: ____________________

Group	Fruits	Vegetables	Grains	Meat & Beans	Milk	Oils
Goal Amount						
Estimate Your Total						
Increase ⇧ or Decrease? ⇩						

Physical Activity: ____________________ Spiritual Activity: ____________________

Steps/Miles/Minutes: ____________________

Day/Date: _____

Breakfast: _____ Lunch: _____
_____
Dinner: _____ Snack: _____
_____

Group	Fruits	Vegetables	Grains	Meat & Beans	Milk	Oils
Goal Amount						
Estimate Your Total						
Increase ⬆ or Decrease? ⬇						

Physical Activity: _____ Spiritual Activity: _____
Steps/Miles/Minutes: _____ _____

Day/Date: _____

Breakfast: _____ Lunch: _____
_____
Dinner: _____ Snack: _____
_____

Group	Fruits	Vegetables	Grains	Meat & Beans	Milk	Oils
Goal Amount						
Estimate Your Total						
Increase ⬆ or Decrease? ⬇						

Physical Activity: _____ Spiritual Activity: _____
Steps/Miles/Minutes: _____ _____

Day/Date: _____

Breakfast: _____ Lunch: _____
_____
Dinner: _____ Snack: _____
_____

Group	Fruits	Vegetables	Grains	Meat & Beans	Milk	Oils
Goal Amount						
Estimate Your Total						
Increase ⬆ or Decrease? ⬇						

Physical Activity: _____ Spiritual Activity: _____
Steps/Miles/Minutes: _____ _____

Day/Date: _____

Breakfast: _____ Lunch: _____
_____
Dinner: _____ Snack: _____
_____

Group	Fruits	Vegetables	Grains	Meat & Beans	Milk	Oils
Goal Amount						
Estimate Your Total						
Increase ⬆ or Decrease? ⬇						

Physical Activity: _____ Spiritual Activity: _____
Steps/Miles/Minutes: _____ _____

Live It Tracker

Name: _____ Loss/gain: _____ lbs.

Date: _____ Week #: _____ Calorie Range: _____ My food goal for next week: _____

Activity Level: None, < 30 min/day, 30-60 min/day, 60+ min/day My activity goal for next week: _____

Group	Daily Calories							
	1300-1400	1500-1600	1700-1800	1900-2000	2100-2200	2300-2400	2500-2600	2700-2800
Fruits	1.5-2 c.	1.5-2 c.	1.5-2 c.	2-2.5 c.	2-2.5 c.	2.5-3.5 c.	3.5-4.5 c.	3.5-4.5 c.
Vegetables	1.5-2 c.	2-2.5 c.	2.5-3 c.	2.5-3 c.	3-3.5 c.	3.5-4.5 c.	4.5-5 c.	4.5-5 c.
Grains	5 oz-eq.	5-6 oz-eq.	6-7 oz-eq.	6-7 oz-eq.	7-8 oz-eq.	8-9 oz-eq.	9-10 oz-eq.	10-11 oz-eq.
Meat & Beans	4 oz-eq.	5 oz-eq.	5-5.5 oz-eq.	5.5-6.5 oz-eq.	6.5-7 oz-eq.	7-7.5 oz-eq.	7-7.5 oz-eq.	7.5-8 oz-eq.
Milk	2-3 c.	3 c.	3 c.	3 c.	3 c.	3 c.	3 c.	3 c.
Healthy Oils	4 tsp.	5 tsp.	5 tsp.	6 tsp.	6 tsp.	7 tsp.	8 tsp.	8 tsp.

Day/Date: _____

Breakfast: _____ Lunch: _____

Dinner: _____ Snack: _____

Group	Fruits	Vegetables	Grains	Meat & Beans	Milk	Oils
Goal Amount						
Estimate Your Total						
Increase ⇧ or Decrease? ⇩						

Physical Activity: _____ Spiritual Activity: _____

Steps/Miles/Minutes: _____ _____

Day/Date: _____

Breakfast: _____ Lunch: _____

Dinner: _____ Snack: _____

Group	Fruits	Vegetables	Grains	Meat & Beans	Milk	Oils
Goal Amount						
Estimate Your Total						
Increase ⇧ or Decrease? ⇩						

Physical Activity: _____ Spiritual Activity: _____

Steps/Miles/Minutes: _____ _____

Day/Date: _____

Breakfast: _____ Lunch: _____

Dinner: _____ Snack: _____

Group	Fruits	Vegetables	Grains	Meat & Beans	Milk	Oils
Goal Amount						
Estimate Your Total						
Increase ⇧ or Decrease? ⇩						

Physical Activity: _____ Spiritual Activity: _____

Steps/Miles/Minutes: _____

Day/Date: _____

Breakfast: _____   Lunch: _____

Dinner: _____   Snack: _____

Group	Fruits	Vegetables	Grains	Meat & Beans	Milk	Oils
Goal Amount						
Estimate Your Total						
Increase ⇧ or Decrease? ⇩						

Physical Activity: _____   Spiritual Activity: _____

Steps/Miles/Minutes: _____   _____

Day/Date: _____

Breakfast: _____   Lunch: _____

Dinner: _____   Snack: _____

Group	Fruits	Vegetables	Grains	Meat & Beans	Milk	Oils
Goal Amount						
Estimate Your Total						
Increase ⇧ or Decrease? ⇩						

Physical Activity: _____   Spiritual Activity: _____

Steps/Miles/Minutes: _____   _____

Day/Date: _____

Breakfast: _____   Lunch: _____

Dinner: _____   Snack: _____

Group	Fruits	Vegetables	Grains	Meat & Beans	Milk	Oils
Goal Amount						
Estimate Your Total						
Increase ⇧ or Decrease? ⇩						

Physical Activity: _____   Spiritual Activity: _____

Steps/Miles/Minutes: _____   _____

Day/Date: _____

Breakfast: _____   Lunch: _____

Dinner: _____   Snack: _____

Group	Fruits	Vegetables	Grains	Meat & Beans	Milk	Oils
Goal Amount						
Estimate Your Total						
Increase ⇧ or Decrease? ⇩						

Physical Activity: _____   Spiritual Activity: _____

Steps/Miles/Minutes: _____   _____

Live It Tracker

Name: _____ Loss/gain: _____ lbs.

Date: _____ Week #: _____ Calorie Range: _____ My food goal for next week: _____

Activity Level: None, < 30 min/day, 30-60 min/day, 60+ min/day My activity goal for next week: _____

Group	Daily Calories							
	1300-1400	1500-1600	1700-1800	1900-2000	2100-2200	2300-2400	2500-2600	2700-2800
Fruits	1.5-2 c.	1.5-2 c.	1.5-2 c.	2-2.5 c.	2-2.5 c.	2.5-3.5 c.	3.5-4.5 c.	3.5-4.5 c.
Vegetables	1.5-2 c.	2-2.5 c.	2.5-3 c.	2.5-3 c.	3-3.5 c.	3.5-4.5 c.	4.5-5 c.	4.5-5 c.
Grains	5 oz-eq.	5-6 oz-eq.	6-7 oz-eq.	6-7 oz-eq.	7-8 oz-eq.	8-9 oz-eq.	9-10 oz-eq.	10-11 oz-eq.
Meat & Beans	4 oz-eq.	5 oz-eq.	5-5.5 oz-eq.	5.5-6.5 oz-eq.	6.5-7 oz-eq.	7-7.5 oz-eq.	7-7.5 oz-eq.	7.5-8 oz-eq.
Milk	2-3 c.	3 c.	3 c.	3 c.	3 c.	3 c.	3 c.	3 c.
Healthy Oils	4 tsp.	5 tsp.	5 tsp.	6 tsp.	6 tsp.	7 tsp.	8 tsp.	8 tsp.

Day/Date:

Breakfast: _____ Lunch: _____

Dinner: _____ Snack: _____

Group	Fruits	Vegetables	Grains	Meat & Beans	Milk	Oils
Goal Amount						
Estimate Your Total						
Increase ⇧ or Decrease? ⇩						

Physical Activity: _____ Spiritual Activity: _____

Steps/Miles/Minutes: _____

Day/Date:

Breakfast: _____ Lunch: _____

Dinner: _____ Snack: _____

Group	Fruits	Vegetables	Grains	Meat & Beans	Milk	Oils
Goal Amount						
Estimate Your Total						
Increase ⇧ or Decrease? ⇩						

Physical Activity: _____ Spiritual Activity: _____

Steps/Miles/Minutes: _____

Day/Date:

Breakfast: _____ Lunch: _____

Dinner: _____ Snack: _____

Group	Fruits	Vegetables	Grains	Meat & Beans	Milk	Oils
Goal Amount						
Estimate Your Total						
Increase ⇧ or Decrease? ⇩						

Physical Activity: _____ Spiritual Activity: _____

Steps/Miles/Minutes: _____

Day/Date: ___

Breakfast: _____   Lunch: _____
_____   _____
Dinner: _____   Snack: _____
_____   _____

Group	Fruits	Vegetables	Grains	Meat & Beans	Milk	Oils
Goal Amount						
Estimate Your Total						
Increase ⇧ or Decrease? ⇩						

Physical Activity: _____   Spiritual Activity: _____
Steps/Miles/Minutes: _____   _____

Day/Date: ___

Breakfast: _____   Lunch: _____
_____   _____
Dinner: _____   Snack: _____
_____   _____

Group	Fruits	Vegetables	Grains	Meat & Beans	Milk	Oils
Goal Amount						
Estimate Your Total						
Increase ⇧ or Decrease? ⇩						

Physical Activity: _____   Spiritual Activity: _____
Steps/Miles/Minutes: _____   _____

Day/Date: ___

Breakfast: _____   Lunch: _____
_____   _____
Dinner: _____   Snack: _____
_____   _____

Group	Fruits	Vegetables	Grains	Meat & Beans	Milk	Oils
Goal Amount						
Estimate Your Total						
Increase ⇧ or Decrease? ⇩						

Physical Activity: _____   Spiritual Activity: _____
Steps/Miles/Minutes: _____   _____

Day/Date: ___

Breakfast: _____   Lunch: _____
_____   _____
Dinner: _____   Snack: _____
_____   _____

Group	Fruits	Vegetables	Grains	Meat & Beans	Milk	Oils
Goal Amount						
Estimate Your Total						
Increase ⇧ or Decrease? ⇩						

Physical Activity: _____   Spiritual Activity: _____
Steps/Miles/Minutes: _____   _____

Live It Tracker

Name: _____ Loss/gain: _____ lbs.

Date: _____ Week #: _____ Calorie Range: _____ My food goal for next week: _____

Activity Level: None, < 30 min/day, 30-60 min/day, 60+ min/day My activity goal for next week: _____

Group	Daily Calories							
	1300-1400	1500-1600	1700-1800	1900-2000	2100-2200	2300-2400	2500-2600	2700-2800
Fruits	1.5-2 c.	1.5-2 c.	1.5-2 c.	2-2.5 c.	2-2.5 c.	2.5-3.5 c.	3.5-4.5 c.	3.5-4.5 c.
Vegetables	1.5-2 c.	2-2.5 c.	2.5-3 c.	2.5-3 c.	3-3.5 c.	3.5-4.5 c.	4.5-5 c.	4.5-5 c.
Grains	5 oz-eq.	5-6 oz-eq.	6-7 oz-eq.	6-7 oz-eq.	7-8 oz-eq.	8-9 oz-eq.	9-10 oz-eq.	10-11 oz-eq.
Meat & Beans	4 oz-eq.	5 oz-eq.	5-5.5 oz-eq.	5.5-6.5 oz-eq.	6.5-7 oz-eq.	7-7.5 oz-eq.	7-7.5 oz-eq.	7.5-8 oz-eq.
Milk	2-3 c.	3 c.	3 c.	3 c.	3 c.	3 c.	3 c.	3 c.
Healthy Oils	4 tsp.	5 tsp.	5 tsp.	6 tsp.	6 tsp.	7 tsp.	8 tsp.	8 tsp.

Day/Date: ____

Breakfast: _____ Lunch: _____

Dinner: _____ Snack: _____

Group	Fruits	Vegetables	Grains	Meat & Beans	Milk	Oils
Goal Amount						
Estimate Your Total						
Increase ⇧ or Decrease? ⇩						

Physical Activity: _____ Spiritual Activity: _____

Steps/Miles/Minutes: _____

Day/Date: ____

Breakfast: _____ Lunch: _____

Dinner: _____ Snack: _____

Group	Fruits	Vegetables	Grains	Meat & Beans	Milk	Oils
Goal Amount						
Estimate Your Total						
Increase ⇧ or Decrease? ⇩						

Physical Activity: _____ Spiritual Activity: _____

Steps/Miles/Minutes: _____

Day/Date: ____

Breakfast: _____ Lunch: _____

Dinner: _____ Snack: _____

Group	Fruits	Vegetables	Grains	Meat & Beans	Milk	Oils
Goal Amount						
Estimate Your Total						
Increase ⇧ or Decrease? ⇩						

Physical Activity: _____ Spiritual Activity: _____

Steps/Miles/Minutes: _____

Day/Date:

Breakfast: _____ Lunch: _____

Dinner: _____ Snack: _____

Group	Fruits	Vegetables	Grains	Meat & Beans	Milk	Oils
Goal Amount						
Estimate Your Total						
Increase ⇧ or Decrease? ⇩						

Physical Activity: _____ Spiritual Activity: _____

Steps/Miles/Minutes: _____ _____

Day/Date:

Breakfast: _____ Lunch: _____

Dinner: _____ Snack: _____

Group	Fruits	Vegetables	Grains	Meat & Beans	Milk	Oils
Goal Amount						
Estimate Your Total						
Increase ⇧ or Decrease? ⇩						

Physical Activity: _____ Spiritual Activity: _____

Steps/Miles/Minutes: _____ _____

Day/Date:

Breakfast: _____ Lunch: _____

Dinner: _____ Snack: _____

Group	Fruits	Vegetables	Grains	Meat & Beans	Milk	Oils
Goal Amount						
Estimate Your Total						
Increase ⇧ or Decrease? ⇩						

Physical Activity: _____ Spiritual Activity: _____

Steps/Miles/Minutes: _____ _____

Day/Date:

Breakfast: _____ Lunch: _____

Dinner: _____ Snack: _____

Group	Fruits	Vegetables	Grains	Meat & Beans	Milk	Oils
Goal Amount						
Estimate Your Total						
Increase ⇧ or Decrease? ⇩						

Physical Activity: _____ Spiritual Activity: _____

Steps/Miles/Minutes: _____ _____

Live It Tracker

Name: _____ Loss/gain: _____ lbs.

Date: _____ Week #: _____ Calorie Range: _____ My food goal for next week: _____

Activity Level: None, < 30 min/day, 30-60 min/day, 60+ min/day My activity goal for next week: _____

Group	Daily Calories							
	1300-1400	1500-1600	1700-1800	1900-2000	2100-2200	2300-2400	2500-2600	2700-2800
Fruits	1.5-2 c.	1.5-2 c.	1.5-2 c.	2-2.5 c.	2-2.5 c.	2.5-3.5 c.	3.5-4.5 c.	3.5-4.5 c.
Vegetables	1.5-2 c.	2-2.5 c.	2.5-3 c.	2.5-3 c.	3-3.5 c.	3.5-4.5 c.	4.5-5 c.	4.5-5 c.
Grains	5 oz-eq.	5-6 oz-eq.	6-7 oz-eq.	6-7 oz-eq.	7-8 oz-eq.	8-9 oz-eq.	9-10 oz-eq.	10-11 oz-eq.
Meat & Beans	4 oz-eq.	5 oz-eq.	5-5.5 oz-eq.	5.5-6.5 oz-eq.	6.5-7 oz-eq.	7-7.5 oz-eq.	7-7.5 oz-eq.	7.5-8 oz-eq.
Milk	2-3 c.	3 c.	3 c.	3 c.	3 c.	3 c.	3 c.	3 c.
Healthy Oils	4 tsp.	5 tsp.	5 tsp.	6 tsp.	6 tsp.	7 tsp.	8 tsp.	8 tsp.

Day/Date: _____

Breakfast: _____   Lunch: _____

Dinner: _____   Snack: _____

Group	Fruits	Vegetables	Grains	Meat & Beans	Milk	Oils
Goal Amount						
Estimate Your Total						
Increase ⇧ or Decrease? ⇩						

Physical Activity: _____   Spiritual Activity: _____

Steps/Miles/Minutes: _____

Day/Date: _____

Breakfast: _____   Lunch: _____

Dinner: _____   Snack: _____

Group	Fruits	Vegetables	Grains	Meat & Beans	Milk	Oils
Goal Amount						
Estimate Your Total						
Increase ⇧ or Decrease? ⇩						

Physical Activity: _____   Spiritual Activity: _____

Steps/Miles/Minutes: _____

Day/Date: _____

Breakfast: _____   Lunch: _____

Dinner: _____   Snack: _____

Group	Fruits	Vegetables	Grains	Meat & Beans	Milk	Oils
Goal Amount						
Estimate Your Total						
Increase ⇧ or Decrease? ⇩						

Physical Activity: _____   Spiritual Activity: _____

Steps/Miles/Minutes: _____

Day/Date: _____

Breakfast: _____ Lunch: _____

Dinner: _____ Snack: _____

Group	Fruits	Vegetables	Grains	Meat & Beans	Milk	Oils
Goal Amount						
Estimate Your Total						
Increase ⇧ or Decrease? ⇩						

Physical Activity: _____ Spiritual Activity: _____

Steps/Miles/Minutes: _____ _____

Day/Date: _____

Breakfast: _____ Lunch: _____

Dinner: _____ Snack: _____

Group	Fruits	Vegetables	Grains	Meat & Beans	Milk	Oils
Goal Amount						
Estimate Your Total						
Increase ⇧ or Decrease? ⇩						

Physical Activity: _____ Spiritual Activity: _____

Steps/Miles/Minutes: _____ _____

Day/Date: _____

Breakfast: _____ Lunch: _____

Dinner: _____ Snack: _____

Group	Fruits	Vegetables	Grains	Meat & Beans	Milk	Oils
Goal Amount						
Estimate Your Total						
Increase ⇧ or Decrease? ⇩						

Physical Activity: _____ Spiritual Activity: _____

Steps/Miles/Minutes: _____ _____

Day/Date: _____

Breakfast: _____ Lunch: _____

Dinner: _____ Snack: _____

Group	Fruits	Vegetables	Grains	Meat & Beans	Milk	Oils
Goal Amount						
Estimate Your Total						
Increase ⇧ or Decrease? ⇩						

Physical Activity: _____ Spiritual Activity: _____

Steps/Miles/Minutes: _____ _____

Live It Tracker

Name: _____ Loss/gain: _____ lbs.

Date: _____ Week #: _____ Calorie Range: _____ My food goal for next week: _____

Activity Level: None, < 30 min/day, 30-60 min/day, 60+ min/day My activity goal for next week: _____

Group	Daily Calories							
	1300-1400	1500-1600	1700-1800	1900-2000	2100-2200	2300-2400	2500-2600	2700-2800
Fruits	1.5-2 c.	1.5-2 c.	1.5-2 c.	2-2.5 c.	2-2.5 c.	2.5-3.5 c.	3.5-4.5 c.	3.5-4.5 c.
Vegetables	1.5-2 c.	2-2.5 c.	2.5-3 c.	2.5-3 c.	3-3.5 c.	3.5-4.5 c.	4.5-5 c.	4.5-5 c.
Grains	5 oz-eq.	5-6 oz-eq.	6-7 oz-eq.	6-7 oz-eq.	7-8 oz-eq.	8-9 oz-eq.	9-10 oz-eq.	10-11 oz-eq.
Meat & Beans	4 oz-eq.	5 oz-eq.	5-5.5 oz-eq.	5.5-6.5 oz-eq.	6.5-7 oz-eq.	7-7.5 oz-eq.	7-7.5 oz-eq.	7.5-8 oz-eq.
Milk	2-3 c.	3 c.	3 c.	3 c.	3 c.	3 c.	3 c.	3 c.
Healthy Oils	4 tsp.	5 tsp.	5 tsp.	6 tsp.	6 tsp.	7 tsp.	8 tsp.	8 tsp.

Day/Date: _____

Breakfast: _____   Lunch: _____

Dinner: _____   Snack: _____

Group	Fruits	Vegetables	Grains	Meat & Beans	Milk	Oils
Goal Amount						
Estimate Your Total						
Increase ⇧ or Decrease? ⇩						

Physical Activity: _____   Spiritual Activity: _____

Steps/Miles/Minutes: _____

Day/Date: _____

Breakfast: _____   Lunch: _____

Dinner: _____   Snack: _____

Group	Fruits	Vegetables	Grains	Meat & Beans	Milk	Oils
Goal Amount						
Estimate Your Total						
Increase ⇧ or Decrease? ⇩						

Physical Activity: _____   Spiritual Activity: _____

Steps/Miles/Minutes: _____

Day/Date: _____

Breakfast: _____   Lunch: _____

Dinner: _____   Snack: _____

Group	Fruits	Vegetables	Grains	Meat & Beans	Milk	Oils
Goal Amount						
Estimate Your Total						
Increase ⇧ or Decrease? ⇩						

Physical Activity: _____   Spiritual Activity: _____

Steps/Miles/Minutes: _____

Day/Date:

Breakfast: _____ Lunch: _____

Dinner: _____ Snack: _____

Group	Fruits	Vegetables	Grains	Meat & Beans	Milk	Oils
Goal Amount						
Estimate Your Total						
Increase ⬆ or Decrease? ⬇						

Physical Activity: _____ Spiritual Activity: _____

Steps/Miles/Minutes: _____ _____

Day/Date:

Breakfast: _____ Lunch: _____

Dinner: _____ Snack: _____

Group	Fruits	Vegetables	Grains	Meat & Beans	Milk	Oils
Goal Amount						
Estimate Your Total						
Increase ⬆ or Decrease? ⬇						

Physical Activity: _____ Spiritual Activity: _____

Steps/Miles/Minutes: _____ _____

Day/Date:

Breakfast: _____ Lunch: _____

Dinner: _____ Snack: _____

Group	Fruits	Vegetables	Grains	Meat & Beans	Milk	Oils
Goal Amount						
Estimate Your Total						
Increase ⬆ or Decrease? ⬇						

Physical Activity: _____ Spiritual Activity: _____

Steps/Miles/Minutes: _____ _____

Day/Date:

Breakfast: _____ Lunch: _____

Dinner: _____ Snack: _____

Group	Fruits	Vegetables	Grains	Meat & Beans	Milk	Oils
Goal Amount						
Estimate Your Total						
Increase ⬆ or Decrease? ⬇						

Physical Activity: _____ Spiritual Activity: _____

Steps/Miles/Minutes: _____ _____

Live It Tracker

Name: _____ Loss/gain: _____ lbs.

Date: _____ Week #: _____ Calorie Range: _____ My food goal for next week: _____

Activity Level: None, < 30 min/day, 30-60 min/day, 60+ min/day   My activity goal for next week: _____

Group	Daily Calories							
	1300-1400	1500-1600	1700-1800	1900-2000	2100-2200	2300-2400	2500-2600	2700-2800
Fruits	1.5-2 c.	1.5-2 c.	1.5-2 c.	2-2.5 c.	2-2.5 c.	2.5-3.5 c.	3.5-4.5 c.	3.5-4.5 c.
Vegetables	1.5-2 c.	2-2.5 c.	2.5-3 c.	2.5-3 c.	3-3.5 c.	3.5-4.5 c.	4.5-5 c.	4.5-5 c.
Grains	5 oz-eq.	5-6 oz-eq.	6-7 oz-eq.	6-7 oz-eq.	7-8 oz-eq.	8-9 oz-eq.	9-10 oz-eq.	10-11 oz-eq.
Meat & Beans	4 oz-eq.	5 oz-eq.	5-5.5 oz-eq.	5.5-6.5 oz-eq.	6.5-7 oz-eq.	7-7.5 oz-eq.	7-7.5 oz-eq.	7.5-8 oz-eq.
Milk	2-3 c.	3 c.	3 c.	3 c.	3 c.	3 c.	3 c.	3 c.
Healthy Oils	4 tsp.	5 tsp.	5 tsp.	6 tsp.	6 tsp.	7 tsp.	8 tsp.	8 tsp.

Day/Date: _____

Breakfast: _____   Lunch: _____

Dinner: _____   Snack: _____

Group	Fruits	Vegetables	Grains	Meat & Beans	Milk	Oils
Goal Amount						
Estimate Your Total						
Increase ⇧ or Decrease? ⇩						

Physical Activity: _____   Spiritual Activity: _____

Steps/Miles/Minutes: _____

Day/Date: _____

Breakfast: _____   Lunch: _____

Dinner: _____   Snack: _____

Group	Fruits	Vegetables	Grains	Meat & Beans	Milk	Oils
Goal Amount						
Estimate Your Total						
Increase ⇧ or Decrease? ⇩						

Physical Activity: _____   Spiritual Activity: _____

Steps/Miles/Minutes: _____

Day/Date: _____

Breakfast: _____   Lunch: _____

Dinner: _____   Snack: _____

Group	Fruits	Vegetables	Grains	Meat & Beans	Milk	Oils
Goal Amount						
Estimate Your Total						
Increase ⇧ or Decrease? ⇩						

Physical Activity: _____   Spiritual Activity: _____

Steps/Miles/Minutes: _____

Day/Date:

Breakfast: _____   Lunch: _____
_____   _____
Dinner: _____   Snack: _____
_____   _____

Group	Fruits	Vegetables	Grains	Meat & Beans	Milk	Oils
Goal Amount						
Estimate Your Total						
Increase ⇧ or Decrease? ⇩						

Physical Activity: _____   Spiritual Activity: _____
Steps/Miles/Minutes: _____   _____

Day/Date:

Breakfast: _____   Lunch: _____
_____   _____
Dinner: _____   Snack: _____
_____   _____

Group	Fruits	Vegetables	Grains	Meat & Beans	Milk	Oils
Goal Amount						
Estimate Your Total						
Increase ⇧ or Decrease? ⇩						

Physical Activity: _____   Spiritual Activity: _____
Steps/Miles/Minutes: _____   _____

Day/Date:

Breakfast: _____   Lunch: _____
_____   _____
Dinner: _____   Snack: _____
_____   _____

Group	Fruits	Vegetables	Grains	Meat & Beans	Milk	Oils
Goal Amount						
Estimate Your Total						
Increase ⇧ or Decrease? ⇩						

Physical Activity: _____   Spiritual Activity: _____
Steps/Miles/Minutes: _____   _____

Day/Date:

Breakfast: _____   Lunch: _____
_____   _____
Dinner: _____   Snack: _____
_____   _____

Group	Fruits	Vegetables	Grains	Meat & Beans	Milk	Oils
Goal Amount						
Estimate Your Total						
Increase ⇧ or Decrease? ⇩						

Physical Activity: _____   Spiritual Activity: _____
Steps/Miles/Minutes: _____   _____

let's count our miles!

Join the 100-Mile Club this Session

Can't walk that mile yet? Don't be discouraged! There are exercises you can do to strengthen your body and burn those extra calories. Keep a record on your Live It Tracker of the number of minutes you do these common physical activities, convert those minutes to miles following the chart below, and then mark off each mile you have completed on the chart found on the back of the front cover. Report your miles to your 100-Mile Club representative when you first arrive each week. Remember, you are not competing with anyone else . . . just yourself. Your job is to strive to reach 100 miles before the last meeting in this session. You can do it—just keep on moving!

Walking

slowly, 2 mph	30 min. = 156 cal. = 1 mile
moderately, 3 mph	20 min. = 156 cal. = 1 mile
very briskly, 4 mph	15 min. = 156 cal. = 1 mile
speed walking	10 min. = 156 cal. = 1 mile
up stairs	13 min. = 159 cal. = 1 mile

Running/Jogging
10 min. = 156 cal. = 1 mile

Cycling Outdoors

slowly, <10 mph	20 min. = 156 cal. = 1 mile
light effort, 10-12 mph	12 min. = 156 cal. = 1 mile
moderate effort, 12-14 mph.	10 min. = 156 cal. = 1 mile
vigorous effort, 14-16 mph	7.5 min. = 156 cal. = 1 mile
very fast, 16-19 mph	6.5 min. = 152 cal. = 1 mile

Sports Activities

Playing tennis (singles)	10 min. = 156 cal. = 1 mile
Swimming	
light to moderate effort	11 min. = 152 cal. = 1 mile
fast, vigorous effort	7.5 min. = 156 cal. = 1 mile
Softball	15 min. = 156 cal. = 1 mile
Golf	20 min. = 156 cal = 1 mile
Rollerblading	6.5 min. = 152 cal. = 1 mile
Ice skating	11 min. = 152 cal. = 1 mile

Jumping rope	7.5 min. = 156 cal. = 1 mile
Basketball	12 min. = 156 cal. = 1 mile
Soccer (casual)	15 min. = 159 cal. = 1 mile

Around the House

Mowing grass	22 min. = 156 cal. = 1 mile
Mopping, sweeping, vacuuming	19.5 min. = 155 cal. = 1 mile
Cooking	40 min. =160 cal. = 1 mile
Gardening	19 min. = 156 cal. = 1 mile
Housework (general)	35 min. = 156 cal. = 1 mile
Ironing	45 min. = 153 cal. = 1 mile
Raking leaves	25 min. = 150 cal. = 1 mile
Washing car	23 min. = 156 cal. = 1 mile
Washing dishes	45 min. = 153 cal. = 1 mile

At the Gym

Stair machine	8.5 min. = 155 cal. = 1 mile
Stationary bike	
slowly, 10 mph	30 min. = 156 cal. = 1 mile
moderately, 10-13 mph	15 min. = 156 cal. = 1 mile
vigorously, 13-16 mph	7.5 min. = 156 cal. = 1 mile
briskly, 16-19 mph	6.5 min. = 156 cal. = 1 mile
Elliptical trainer	12 min. = 156 cal. = 1 mile
Weight machines (used vigorously)	13 min. = 152 cal.=1 mile
Aerobics	
low impact	15 min. = 156 cal. = 1 mile
high impact	12 min. = 156 cal. = 1 mile
water	20 min. = 156 cal. = 1 mile
Pilates	15 min. = 156 cal. = 1 mile
Raquetball (casual)	15 min. = 159 cal. = 1 mile
Stretching exercises	25 min. = 150 cal. = 1 mile
Weight lifting (also works for weight machines used moderately or gently)	30 min. = 156 cal. = 1 mile

Family Leisure

Playing piano	37 min. = 155 cal. = 1 mile
Jumping rope	10 min. = 152 cal. = 1 mile
Skating (moderate)	20 min. = 152 cal. = 1 mile
Swimming	
moderate	17 min. = 156 cal. = 1 mile
vigorous	10 min. = 148 cal. = 1 mile
Table tennis	25 min. = 150 cal. = 1 mile
Walk/run/play with kids	25 min. = 150 cal. = 1 mile